DUMB BELLS & DOPAMINE

PARKINSON'S
SUCCESS STORY

by

Arthur W. Curren

authorHOUSE™

1663 Liberty Drive, Suite 200
Bloomington, Indiana 47403
(800) 839-8640
www.AuthorHouse.com

First published by AuthorHouse 12/21/2005

ISBN: 1-4259-0185-9 (sc)

Library of Congress Control Number: 2005910773

Printed in the United States of America
Bloomington, Indiana

The author believes that his combination of a rigorous exercise routine and the prudent use of the available drugs has enabled him to retard the advance of his Parkinson's disease. The author also believes that most of the people with Parkinson's who can follow a similar exercise routine and drug regimen will be able to retard the advance of the disease. However, because of the variations within the disease, it is unrealistic to expect that all of the people who follow his dumb bells and dopamine concept will be successful.

People with Parkinson's who have physical problems other than those related to Parkinson's disease should not attempt to participate in the exercise routine described in this book without the approval of the appropriate health care professional. People with Parkinson's who cannot perform an exercise or exercises correctly without dumb bells, should not attempt to perform the exercise or exercises with dumb bells.

This book is printed on acid-free paper.

This book is dedicated to my father, Wallace Curren, from whom I inherited the stubborn streak that makes living with Parkinson's disease a little more tolerable.

Acknowledgments

The author wishes to acknowledge the assistance of those who played a major role in the production of this book:

To Andrew Gray of the Department of Theatre, Film and Creative Writing at the University of British Columbia, for his guidance during the early development of the book;

To my sister Anna and daughter Carol for their help during the development of the text, with their many suggestions and corrections to the manuscript;

To my son Richard for the design and production of the covers and illustrations;

To my wife Sheila for coordinating the whole thing to produce the finished product.

Foreword

Parkinson's is a debilitating disease for which there is no cure. People with the disease are in a no-win situation where success has to be measured with a very different yardstick. That yardstick is the measure of a person's ability to retard the advance of the disease.

In that regard I have achieved a level of success because after more than twenty years with the disease I can easily perform all of the day-to-day requirements of life without any assistance from others. There are not a lot of people with Parkinson's who can make that statement.

To understand the issues involved in living with Parkinson's I have included a detailed description of the disease as well as the treatment options that are available. I have also provided details of the therapies that I chose to follow. I believe that most of my success with the disease has been the result of a rigorous exercise routine together with the prudent use of the available drugs. I also believe that a no-quit stubborn streak that I inherited from my father has been a positive factor in my struggle with the disease.

In addition to the day-to-day issues of living with the disease, I had to deal with problems that were created by the fact that I had Parkinson's. I was blacklisted by the insurance industry and denied Social Security disability benefits. I was also used and abused by incompetent and dishonest physicians. All of those issues made life interesting and are covered in detail.

To obtain employment and remain employed, it was necessary for me to hide the fact that I had Parkinson's disease. To accomplish that goal I had to find ways to hide the symptoms of the disease. That deception, together with the help of a few co-workers who looked the other way, enabled me to stay employed for more than a decade after the onset of the disease.

It seems that all prescription drugs have at least two names. The medications approved for Parkinson's are no exception. Deprenyl for instance has at least three names. In an attempt to reduce the confusion I have chosen to refer to all of the Parkinson's drugs by the names they were assigned when they were first manufactured. The various trade or brand names and the generic names of the Parkinson's medications that I have used are listed in the appendix.

In order to avoid the possibility of being involved in groundless, unfriendly litigation, the names of all of the medical practitioners whom I encountered were changed. Any similarity of the assumed names to persons living or dead would be entirely coincidental. Dr. Morton Shulman and Dr. Malcolm Sayer, whom I did not encounter, are referred to by their correct names.

Table of Contents

PART ONE

Beginning the Story: Early Symptoms

1. The Tip of the Iceberg

"You're really slapping that foot tonight." That astute comment came from my running mate and as usual she was right. For the past year or so I had trouble controlling my left foot when running. Tonight it was worse than usual.

It was a summer evening in 1982 and we were in Friendswood, Texas, a suburb of Houston. We were about halfway through a two mile run. The pattern was the same. My left leg would tire before the right and I would lose a measure of control over the functioning of my left foot. The smooth transition of motion from heel to toe was missing. It had been replaced by an uncontrolled transition where heel contact was followed by the ball of the foot slapping the pavement.

I had been running for about seventeen years. I had run through shin splints, bone bruises and other assorted aches and pains that plague distance runners. They all hurt and they all took time to heal. This problem seemed to be different in that it was not one of the things that a runner could expect to encounter. Also it was not getting any better.

Other problems were starting to emerge. I had been actively involved in weight training since my late teens, a period of some thirty-two years. For about thirty of those years I had been pumping iron without any significant movement of the unsecured plates that I had stacked on each end of the barbell. The exercises that I used to perform smoothly were now being done in a way that caused some of the plates to rattle. I tried reducing the weights but the rattle was still there. I was then in my fiftieth year and I thought it might be due to aging, but as it continued to worsen I began to wonder.

I was also starting to have problems in everyday life. Controlling a bar of soap while taking a shower was becoming difficult. Using a fork and knife when eating required an increased level of concentration. My handwriting, which at best was marginal, now required increased concentration just to make it readable. I was able to rationalize things away for a while but eventually I had to face reality. I had to accept the fact that I had a problem that was getting worse and was not going to go away.

Mohammed Ali was no longer the heavyweight champion but he still claimed to be the greatest. Michael J. Fox had yet to go "Back to the Future." In fact it would be about two years before he would make that movie. At that time virtually no one, myself included, had ever heard of Parkinson's disease.

The problems that I was experiencing in the summer of 1982 were merely the tip of the iceberg. Things were going to get a lot worse. I had Parkinson's disease, but it would be almost five years before I would be diagnosed as having that debilitating disease. In the interim I was to discover that things do not always turn out as expected. The first step in my battle with Parkinson's began with…

2. The Wrong Diagnosis

It was time to accept the fact that my body, or more specifically the muscles of my body, were no longer functioning properly. It was obvious that I was having a problem with my control systems. I further reasoned that because my problem seemed to lie somewhere in my central nervous system I would need the services of a neurologist. The next step was to have a family member or friend recommend a suitable practitioner. Unfortunately that tack yielded nothing and I was forced to consult that bastion of western civilization: the yellow pages.

My initial perusal of that publication indicated that the medical profession had not neglected Houston. The list of neurologists, which seemed to be excessive, contained about forty names. That led to my next problem, how to pick a winner. Based on the assumption that my problem was not some rare, exotic disease, I assumed that any qualified physician would suffice. It therefore followed that I should select the person who was most conveniently located with respect to my home and my work. That selection process led to an appointment with Dr. Evelyn Timmons, a neurologist.

Dr. Timmons was a pleasant woman who appeared to be in her mid-thirties. She listened as I described the problems I was having and asked a number of questions related to those problems. She also asked a number of questions related to my personal history, which included my parents and other family members.

She then conducted a basic neurological examination consisting of a number of simple tests to assess the functioning of my nervous system. My tendon reflexes were evaluated when my knees and ankles were hit with a rubber hammer. Hand, arm and leg strengths were tested to detect muscle weakness. My sensory functions were evaluated by observing my ability to feel pain, heat and cold. The soles of my feet and the palms of my hands were touched with a sharp object to induce pain. A tuning fork was used to test my ability to feel vibrations. I was not surprised to learn that her examination did not detect any major malfunctions or a life threatening disease.

After some consideration she explained that my problems were due to the onset of a disorder known as essential tremor. She described this condition as a rhythmic shaking that usually appears initially in the hands. Over time the tremor may affect the arms and other parts of the body. She said that I was displaying an indication of the beginning of hand tremor. I was vaguely aware of the occasional shaking of a hand from time to time, but because it was barely noticeable I did not consider it to be a real problem.

Dr. Timmons stated that the cause of essential tremor was unknown, and there was no treatment or cure. She further explained that the level of my affliction was considered to be harmless, and her complete diagnosis was "benign essential tremor." I did not entirely believe her because it did not explain the various coordination problems that I was experiencing. There did not seem to be any urgency to get a second opinion, so I decided to let the matter rest for the present.

As my knowledge of the disease increased I was to learn that she missed the mark rather badly. Parkinson's is sometimes diagnosed as essential tremor because the symptoms are similar, especially in the early stages. The most significant difference between Parkinson's and essential tremor lies in the type of tremor that is encountered. With essential tremor the tremor is continuous in that the hand, for instance, shakes when it is at rest and when it is in motion. With Parkinson's the tremor is described as a resting tremor. It occurs when the affected body part is at rest, but not when it is in motion. The hand for instance would be shaking when it is at rest, but would not be shaking when it is in motion.

My tremor, what there was of it, was a resting tremor. The foot slapping that I experienced when running indicated a coordination problem that is sometimes a symptom of Parkinson's disease. It is possible that Dr. Timmons missed my running problem because few, if any, of her patients were runners. However it is difficult to understand how a board-certified neurologist could have missed my resting tremor and obvious coordination problems.

At that time I was employed as a mechanical engineer. I had moved to Houston from California in 1978 to work on a design of synthetic fuel plants that would convert coal and oil shale into products such as gasoline and heating oil. The goal at that time was to achieve energy independence and eliminate our dependence on foreign oil imports. Coal and oil shale deposits in the western states were believed to have the potential to achieve that goal.

Unfortunately the economics of the situation determined that the cost of synthetic fuels was going to be considerably higher than the cost of fuels derived from foreign oil. Coal and oil shale projects that had been started were abruptly cancelled. Houston, that had become the energy capital of the world, saw its economy go from boom to bust.

At the beginning of 1983, at fifty years of age, with my nervous system starting to unravel, my medical problems were abruptly pushed to the back burner. The collapse of Houston's energy based economy impacted my employer and I suddenly found myself unemployed and without health insurance. My physical problems were not yet apparent to family or friends so I decided to hunker down and wait for better days. It was time to enter…

PART TWO

Hard Times in Houston Town: Symptoms Worsen

3. The Survival Mode

My addition to the ranks of the unemployed in the first part of 1983 went completely unnoticed. I was just one among many. It was not just engineering companies that were shedding workers. Companies engaged in related industries such as manufacturing and construction were also victimized by the economic conditions. The ripple effect extended in a lesser degree to unrelated areas such as retailing and real estate. All sorts of people were walking around Houston looking for work. Little did I realize that in spite of my best efforts I would not be able to get a real job until September of 1986.

With absolutely no prospects of employment of any sort I decided that it was time to visit the Texas Employment Commission (TEC) and apply for benefits. Unfortunately my first visit was on a Monday when most of the people who had been terminated the previous Friday descended on the local office. It was mid-morning and the office was full of people, with dozens more milling about outside.

It was my first experience as an unemployed person seeking benefits, and I was surprised at the mood of the crowd. Some people seemed to be in a state of shock, but for the most part the mood could be described as festive. In fact it looked a little like a clambake where somebody was giving away free beer. The situation clearly exceeded the capacity of the TEC office, as there was no way that all of the applicants could be processed in one day. I decided that things could wait a few days and made a mental note to make future visits near the end of the week.

My employment history and related contributions qualified me for maximum benefits. Unfortunately, with a wife and three kids, the TEC benefits fell well short of my expenses. It was obvious that I was going to have to find an additional source of income or my savings would take a big-time hit. With thousands of people unemployed work of any sort was going to be hard to find.

Engineers who applied for minimum wage jobs heard a new reason for rejection. They were considered to be "over qualified." The plight of the engineering profession became the standing joke around Houston. The most common version asked the question, "How many engineers can you put in a station wagon?" The qualified answer was "two, because they have to leave room for their lawn mowers."

I considered mowing lawns but felt I could do a little better making home repairs. Over the years I had done some remodeling of the homes we owned in California and had developed acceptable handyman skills. I discovered that by placing a small ad in the neighborhood newspaper I was able to pick up a few repair jobs. There was never anything big that brought in real money, but it was usually a welcome change from sitting around the house reading the help-wanted section of the Houston Post.

When I was between part-time engineering jobs, which was most of the time, those repair jobs would help close the gap between income and expenses. I was always somewhat amazed at the trust that those homeowners placed in a total stranger. Almost all of them would give me access to their homes and go to work, leaving me alone to make the repair. I will always be indebted to those people who hired an unemployed engineer to repair something that needed fixing.

After about six months among the ranks of the unemployed it became painfully apparent that I was being rejected from some of the jobs that were available because of my age. At that time I was fifty years old and it had become very obvious that anything over forty-something was not going to sell. I could probably have made a case for age discrimination against some of those would-be employers, but it was neither the time nor the place to engage in a long-drawn-out legal action. I had to do something that would generate income as soon as possible. To get a job of any sort I would have to restructure my resume. I decided that I would have to knock eight years off my age.

Fortunately my physical appearance was such that I could pass for forty-two. My hair, although thin on top, was still brown. The years of physical activity had kept my weight under control, and my undiagnosed Parkinson's tremor could still be masked. Reworking the resume was easy. I simply deleted the first eight years of employment and changed my date of graduation from 1955 to 1963. I felt the date change would not be challenged because I had never known an engineering company to confirm an employee's college education. They usually considered confirmation of college degrees to be a waste of time and money. Job performance was the only standard. If you could do the work you stayed, if not you were replaced by someone who could.

Proof of age presented a different problem. I needed some sort of document that showed my adjusted age. There seemed to be no way that I could fake a birth certificate or a passport, so I decided to take a shot at my Texas driver's license. The challenge there was to change my date of birth from 1932 to 1940. I was able to erase the 32 from a Xerox copy of my license. After several attempts I replaced it with an acceptable 40. I then made copies of my adjusted driver's license, which enabled me to provide a suitable document whenever anyone requested proof of age.

No one ever asked to see my actual driver's license, however I am sure that most of those people suspected I was up to something. The bottom line was that if proof of age was required they were all happy to have a piece of paper in my personnel file that would show that they had followed the proper procedure in my employment process.

The engineering jobs that I was able to get prior to September of 1986, were all low pay and short term. With only one exception they were dull and uninteresting. The one exception was…

4. The NASA Caper

The ad in the Houston Chronicle was for an engineer to work on the design of a trash compactor for the space station. I had never heard of the company that had placed the ad. It was located in Clear Lake so I assumed it provided engineering services to NASA. Clear Lake is located southeast of Houston, and at that time to all intents and purposes, it was NASA. It was home to the space agency, its contractors and most of their employees. Because of its association with NASA, Clear Lake had been insulated from the economic problems that the collapse of the energy industry had inflicted on Houston.

I had no knowledge of trash compactors and had never been associated with the space program. I assumed that a trash compactor for an orbiting space station would be a first of its kind and have little in common with a kitchen compactor.

By that time I had prepared a resume for just about every occasion. For instance, if somebody was looking for an engineer to design process piping systems, I had a resume that highlighted my experience in that field. For the trash compactor I decided that I would use my machine design resume. After some consideration I decided that it was probably worth the cost of a first class stamp to submit an application. The application contained all of my experience in the design of mechanical devices. It was not an impressive document, and after mailing it I wondered if it would not have been smarter to hold onto the first class stamp.

To say that I was surprised to hear from an aerospace company had to be the understatement of the year. An interview and a job offer from a company in the Houston area not involved in the energy business seemed unreal. It was not much of an offer, a temporary position that did not pay a lot. However it did pay considerably more than the benefits that I received from the Texas Employment Commission, so I was darn glad to get it. With a NASA related job I hoped that I had found a safe haven where I could drop anchor until things returned to normal.

My employer turned out to be a small company that designed and manufactured tools and accessories for some of the shuttle missions. Most of their fifty or so employees had been there ten or more years. A lot of them had worked in the aerospace industry all of their lives. I was very impressed by the apparent stability of the company.

It was January of 1986 when I began work. My first day on the job began with a company meeting where it was announced that the president of the company had resigned. His resignation was unexpected and nobody seemed to know what was going on. There were the usual speculations, but no answers. For my part, although I am not normally a superstitious person, I considered it to be a bad omen.

A shuttle launch was scheduled for my second day on the job. Shuttle launches at that time were no longer a big thing to the general public. This particular launch had been postponed five times and the news media had become more impatient with each postponement. Some television news-people were starting to ridicule NASA for their inability to launch. The most caustic reporters at the Cape were asking the question, “When is this turkey going to become an eagle?”

To the extended NASA family in the Clear Lake area a launch was still a very big thing because nearly everyone was involved in some way with the event. My employer was no exception and had television sets located throughout the building so that everyone could see the final countdown and liftoff.

STS Mission 51-L began at 11:38 A.M. EST on January 28, 1986, with ignition and liftoff. At 73 seconds into the flight the space shuttle Challenger disintegrated in a huge fireball. Shock and disbelief reigned as the remains of the shuttle and its seven crewmembers fell into the Atlantic Ocean. While I watched the horrific event I could see my career at NASA disintegrate along with Challenger. With the resignation of the company president on my first day and the loss of the Challenger on my second day I could hardly wait to see what my third day on the job would bring.

I was a little surprised and much relieved to find on the next day that things were more or less back to normal. There was no more talk in the news media about turkeys or eagles and my third day on the job was uneventful. It was obvious that NASA was in for some rough sledding in the months ahead and the future did not look good. The shuttle fleet would certainly be grounded. There would be layoffs, and I would probably once again be on the outside looking in.

A review of launch films showed that the cause of the accident was the failure of the pressure seal in the aft field joint of the right solid rocket booster. At 2.5 seconds after liftoff, black smoke could be seen escaping from the seal. At 58 seconds the smoke had become a flame that impinged on the surface of the external tank which contained liquid hydrogen. At 73 seconds the flame caused the shell of the external tank to fail, igniting the hydrogen. The resulting explosion created the huge fireball that destroyed the Challenger.

The investigation that followed showed that the ambient temperature at the launch pad at liftoff was 36 degrees Fahrenheit, 15 degrees colder than any previous launch. The rubber O-ring gasket in the aft field joint was designed for a minimum temperature of 56 degrees Fahrenheit. On some of the previous shuttle launches in cold weather, NASA had found evidence of leakage at some of the field joints on the solid rocket boosters.

NASA management had approved the launch of the Challenger over the objections of their engineers. Their decision was based on internal politics instead of the safety of the mission. They had rolled the dice and lost.

My hope of having found a safe haven ended with the loss of the Challenger. It would be more than a year before the next shuttle mission. In the interim, pending contracts for the shuttle program were placed on the back burner. Contracts that had been awarded were extended to delay their completion. My brief career in the aerospace industry ended in June. I had survived almost five months after the Challenger disaster, much longer than I had expected.

My undiagnosed Parkinson's was becoming a major problem. My hand tremor was starting to occur at the wrong time and had to be masked. Walking sometimes presented a problem, especially when starting. It was clear that I would need medical attention soon, with or without insurance. Employment prospects in the energy industry in Houston were unchanged, that is to say they were just about non-existent. Fortunately for me there was a new game in town and I was about to find…

5. The Real Deal

After the completion of my aerospace adventure in June of 1986 I was once more in the ranks of the unemployed. It was also the beginning of another summer in Houston with its oppressive heat and humidity. The job market for engineers however, had taken a turn for the better. There was a new player in the field and that player was the Environmental Protection Agency, better know by its initials, the EPA.

The EPA was, and is still, a much-maligned agency. At different times it had been accused of doing too little or too much to protect the quality of air and water. In the summer of 1986 it was the prime mover behind regulations relating to the remediation of hazardous waste sites. For the most part these sites were locations where a manufacturer had allowed hazardous chemicals to pollute the soil and groundwater. Remediation was usually accomplished by removing the contaminated soil and recovering and treating the groundwater. The engineering design services needed to remediate a hazardous waste site included mechanical engineering systems that I was capable of designing.

The EPA was also the prime mover for providing new regulations for hazardous waste storage tank systems. The new regulations required that a storage tank with its related piping and equipment was required to meet new standards to ensure the integrity of the system.

All storage tank systems were to be inspected and certified by a registered professional engineer. The inspection and certification were mechanical engineering activities that I could perform. With well over a thousand tank systems in the Houston area, I could expect that work to last for several years. Thanks to the EPA there were now two places where I could expect to find employment.

I was able to find a significant amount of contract work for the certification of storage tank systems during the summer of 1986. Then in September the Houston Post carried a large ad from a small engineering company that was adding a new department to provide engineering services to the developing hazardous waste industry. To be more precise they wanted to design contaminated groundwater recovery and treatment systems. They were planning to hire a total of eight engineers, two of which were to be mechanical engineers. It looked like a really good prospect so I immediately tailored one of my resumes to suit their needs. I must have done something right, because in less than a week I had an interview and a job.

It was my first real job in over three years. It paid decent money with employee benefits that included health insurance. They had funded the new department for a period of one year, so I could count on a job for at least that period of time. Soon after starting work it became apparent that I was in an unusual situation. For the first time in my life I was working with people who, for the most part, were younger than my adjusted age. In fact I was actually the oldest person, by at least five years, in a company that consisted of about thirty people. I was sailing under false colors because of the age issue and did not want to rock the boat. I therefore felt it would be prudent to settle in a little before exposing my problems to their health insurance carrier.

I still had no idea what the next round with a neurologist would disclose. It was possible that my problem would turn out to be an affliction that could cause my employer to conclude that I was a liability instead of an asset. To reduce the possibility of being considered a liability I needed a cover that would allow me to hide the diagnosis if it became necessary. I decided to dredge up an old back injury that I had incurred in my early teens as the basis for seeking an appointment with a neurologist. Back problems are something that most people relate to and it would be a good cover if the diagnosis disclosed an undesirable condition.

After about a month on the job I felt that I had accumulated enough points to actually make an appointment with a neurologist. Because my condition had worsened considerably I fully expected that my next neurology appointment would provide me with the correct diagnosis. Once again I was to learn that things do not always turn out as expected. Instead of getting an appointment with a neurologist who would diagnose my Parkinson's, what I got was an appointment with…

PART THREE

The Opportunists: Medical Misconduct

6. The Setup Man

My employer's health insurance carrier was a large insurance company. However most of the company's medical needs, including annual medical examinations, were provided by a small association of local doctors. The list of their medical staff included a neurologist, which led to an appointment with Dr. Michael Grifton. Dr. Grifton was a person of average height and weight who appeared to be in his early forties. He listened to my story and asked virtually the same questions that Dr. Timmons had asked. Using a rubber hammer and a tuning fork he made the same basic neurological examination that had been performed by Dr. Timmons. He then asked me to walk across the office, turn and walk back.

At the conclusion of his initial examination he said that he had no opinion as to the cause of my problems. He did not rule out essential tremor. He confirmed that I had a neurological problem but he needed more information to diagnose my condition. He recommended that I begin a program of neurological tests so that he could make an accurate diagnosis. That sounded like an excellent idea because it seemed certain that the rubber hammer and tuning fork thing was not going anywhere.

The first test scheduled by Dr. Grifton was a CT scan. Dr. Grifton did not explain the purpose of the CT scan, other than it was performed to detect abnormalities in the brain. Needless to say I was happy to learn that the test results were negative and did not show any problems. It would be years before I would learn that a computed tomography (CT) scan is a non-invasive x-ray procedure that utilizes an ultra thin x-ray beam. The main advantage of a CT scan over an ordinary x-ray is that it shows soft tissue as well as bone. It is used primarily for brain scans in the detection of tumors, strokes and other problems. It is not used in the diagnosis of Parkinson's disease.

The CT scan was followed by an electromyography (EMG) test. That test used two electrodes to induce an electrical current to stimulate various muscles and detect any malfunctions. A strip chart was used to record the results. This test was also non-invasive until the technician decided to get one final reading using a needle electrode that he inserted into my left biceps. Apart from producing about two yards of strip chart the EMG test did nothing to get to the source of my problem.

I was beginning to get the feeling that Dr. Grifton was not going to make a diagnosis until he had extracted as much money as he could from my insurance company. The EMG test was my first indication that the doctor had ordered something that was a waste of time and money. It seemed obvious to me that my problem was in the control of my muscles rather than in the ability of the individual muscles to respond when stimulated.

For the next test Dr. Grifton decided to investigate the possibility that there might be a spinal cord problem. He explained that while a lower back problem could cause a leg problem such as my foot slap, it could not be the cause of my hand tremor. A spinal cord problem that would cause hand tremor would have to be located in the cervical vertebrae, above the point where the nerves merge into the spinal cord. To cover all of the bases he ordered x-rays of the entire spinal column.

The x-rays of my lower back did not show anything significant. However the x-rays of my upper spine showed calcium deposits inside some of my cervical vertebrae that could be exerting pressure on my spinal cord. It seemed that we were finally getting somewhere. To get a better picture of the situation Dr. Grifton ordered a MRI examination.

Magnetic resonance imaging (MRI) was at that time a relatively new technology that was also non-invasive. It utilizes a magnetic field that responds to the hydrogen content of the various organs of the body, to produce a well-defined picture of the internal structure showing both bone and soft tissue. In my case it clearly showed the calcium deposits inside my cervical vertebrae. Some of the deposits seemed to be distorting the shape of my spinal cord. It seemed to me that we had finally found the cause of my problems.

Dr. Grifton never stated that the calcium deposits were the source of my problems. He simply referred to them as an abnormality that should be corrected. When asked about the origin of the calcium deposits he could only state that the body deposits calcium at the site of an injury as a protective function. I had never had a neck injury, so the calcium deposits were of unknown origin.

Over the years I was to learn that there is no test that can confirm Parkinson's disease. It is a movement disorder and its diagnosis is based on the observation of movements that are beyond the control of the afflicted person. The most common indication of Parkinson's disease is probably hand tremor, the involuntary shaking of one or both hands. Another indication is a person's gait, the way a person walks, with special attention to the swinging of the arms.

There is no way that Dr. Grifton could have failed to notice my hand tremor, which at that time was a well-defined resting tremor. Any doubts he had about a diagnosis of Parkinson's disease should have been dispelled when he had me do my little walk-about in his office. At that time my gait was uneven with a slight hesitation at the start. My arm swing was uncoordinated, slightly out of phase with each step, a typical Parkinson's symptom.

None of the tests Dr. Grifton had ordered were needed. He had ripped off my insurance company for the cost of those unnecessary tests, and for his fees for the related office visits.

Instead of receiving a diagnosis of Parkinson's disease I had been set up for an appointment with…

7. The Specialist

Dr. Grifton arranged an appointment with Dr. Philip Cutler, a neurosurgeon, to deal with the calcium deposits that I had been led to believe were the cause of my problems.

Dr. Cutler was a very intense individual. A hyperactive chain smoker, he seemed unable to sit still. If he was not smoking, he was drumming his fingers on the desktop or beating the carpet with one or both of his feet. I was impressed with the way he virtually consumed the MRI prints that he had received from Dr. Grifton. On the other hand I was concerned about his non-stop display of nervous energy.

He asked a few questions about the problems I had with coordination, running and tremor. He said that he agreed with Dr. Grifton's opinion that the calcium deposits were compressing my spinal cord. The problem could be corrected by removing the backs of some of my cervical vertebrae. The procedure, known as a cervical laminectomy, would allow my spinal cord to decompress. At that point in the discussion he dropped what I assume was the standard joke for the situation. He said that, "If you can't lower the river, raise the bridge." Considering the situation, I found his statement to be somewhat humorous.

After reviewing the MRI prints Dr. Cutler stated that he needed one more test. He needed a myelograph, which he described as a series of x-rays of my spine. These would be taken after a dye had been injected into my spinal cord. It sounded like something out of the nineteenth century. He was asking me to undergo a very invasive procedure to obtain x-ray prints that I felt certain would be inferior to the MRI prints he held in his hands. My arguments against that test were to no avail, and it became clear that he was not going to proceed until he had all the test data he felt he needed. I thought briefly about getting another doctor, but decided that I would probably get the same snow job to have what I considered to be an unnecessary test. Also I needed to get the problem fixed while I still had insurance.

After undergoing a very unpleasant session at the myelography lab, I checked into the hospital on December 18, 1986 for surgery the next morning. I did that with considerable trepidation, as I was not convinced that Dr. Cutler had my best interests at heart. I was not sure that I was doing the right thing as they wheeled me down to the operating room and off-loaded me onto the operating table. I was talking to the anesthesiologist as he was setting up shop, when he told me that Dr. Cutler "sure does a lot of work around here." That was all I needed to hear. It confirmed my concern that the good doctor was more interested in money than in people. With the realization that I had probably made a big mistake I decided that it was time for me to get out of there. Unfortunately before I could move the lights went out.

The next thing I knew I was wide-awake in the recovery room. It seemed that I had been unconscious for only an instant. In reality I had been out for several hours. My throat was so dry that I had trouble breathing. The back of my neck was stiff and sore. I immediately began to check out my moveable parts and found that I could move my arms and legs. In less time than it takes to tell, I had determined that all of my body parts were working. I had survived the operation, and suddenly my future looked to be very, very good.

The surgery had been performed without any problems. Dr. Cutler had removed the backs of my C-4, C-5 and C-6 vertebrae, and part of the back of C-7. After a few days in the hospital I was fitted with a cervical collar, and looking like a whiplash claimant at an insurance hearing, I returned home. About a week after the surgery I was back working mornings. Another week and I was back in harness full time.

About a month after the operation, the optimism over my successful cervical laminectomy was starting to wear more than a little thin. My tremor had increased after the surgery, and was showing no signs of abating. I had started running again but the problem with my left leg remained virtually unchanged. My gait, which had worsened after the surgery, was not getting any better. I was not only disappointed, I was starting to get just a little bit angry.

I waited a few more weeks, hoping things would get a little better. When it became obvious that there was not going to be any improvement I made an appointment with Dr. Cutler. It was time to find out just what was going on.

I do not remember the exact dialogue that occurred at that appointment with Dr. Cutler, but I have a crystal clear memory of the substance of the conversation. It began with my statement that his surgery had done nothing to help any of my problems. His response was that he had been hired to remove the backs of some of my cervical vertebrae, which would allow my spinal cord to decompress. He had done that. If I was still having problems it had to be for some other reason. Resisting the justifiable urge to do him bodily harm, I was able to control my temper and ask him where I could go to get help. He replied that in his opinion the best neurologist in Houston was Dr. Joseph Knowles.

Eventually I was to learn that the mysterious calcium deposits were the result of a condition known as cervical spondylosis. It is usually caused by aging and is common in older people. It is possible that at some time in the future I might have needed a cervical laminectomy but there was no need to have it at that time. There is absolutely no doubt in my mind that Dr. Cutler knew that I had Parkinson's disease and took advantage of the situation to make a quick buck.

Dr. Knowles may very well have been the best neurologist in Houston, because he did not lack for patients. I had to wait over two months for my first appointment. I was also to learn that his rate for an office visit was twenty dollars over what my insurance company would pay. It seemed that if he was not one of the best, then he had been fooling an awful lot of people. After having been used and abused for nearly four years, it seemed that in June of 1987, I was finally going to get…

PART FOUR

Revelation:
The Truth at Last

8. The Correct Diagnosis

"You have Parkinson's disease." That was Dr. Knowles' verdict about five minutes into our first meeting. Before his words had time to sink in he added the reassuring statement, "You are not going to die." I thought about that for a few seconds and assumed that what he meant was that I was not going to die soon. I had no idea what Parkinson's disease was, but I was happy to hear that I was not about to buy the farm.

Dr. Knowles had no trouble reaching his diagnosis. He made a basic neurological examination utilizing what seemed to be the tools of the trade, a rubber hammer and a tuning fork. He asked virtually the same questions that the other neurologists had asked and had me do a little walk-about in his office. When he announced his diagnosis he did so with great certainty. This confirmed my opinion that Dr. Grifton belonged in jail and that Dr. Cutler should be his cellmate.

Dr. Knowles explained that Parkinson's disease was a neurological disorder that afflicted older people, usually those on the wrong side of fifty. It was a progressive disease that worsened over time. It attacked both males and females, as well as people of all races. Its cause was unknown and there was no cure. The disease was inconsistent as it attacked people in different ways. The only help for those with the disease came mostly from a few drugs that had been found to be beneficial in most cases. He explained that with continued use all of the drugs approved for Parkinson's disease would gradually lose their ability to be effective.

To assist in my understanding of the disease Dr. Knowles gave me some booklets that had been published by some of the national Parkinson's organizations. These booklets were designed to help people who were newly diagnosed with Parkinson's deal with the disease. He also gave me a list of books that I should read, and a prescription for artane, a drug that might be helpful.

At the end of the session he opened the bottom drawer of his desk and extracted an application form and a brochure for an experimental drug program known as the DATATOP study. The purpose of the study was to determine if either deprenyl, a drug that was used in Europe to treat people with Parkinson's, or tocopherol, a fat soluble compound in use worldwide, could slow the progression of Parkinson's disease. He felt that I would be a good candidate for that program and would probably benefit from the experience. At that time I was not enraptured with the performance of the medical profession, so I told him that I would think about it.

I was now certain that Dr. Grifton and Dr. Cutler had contrived to have me undergo a needless surgery. I had been used by those less than honest doctors for financial gain at the expense of my insurance company. My thoughts immediately turned to initiating a legal action against them. I had some knowledge of how the legal system works and it was immediately apparent that I would need expert witnesses to prove anything against either doctor. It soon became obvious that the cost of hiring lawyers and finding expert witnesses who would rat out their fellow practitioners would be far beyond my resources. I considered filing a complaint with the applicable regulatory agencies, but finally decided it would only be a waste of good writing paper. Reluctantly I realized that it was best to move on and apply my time and resources to finding a way to live with the disease.

The booklets that I received from Dr. Knowles were helpful in defining the disease and explaining the treatment options. However they were less helpful in alerting me about the problems that I would face with the insurance industry and the Social Security Administration because I had Parkinson's disease.

I planned to read some of the books that Dr. Knowles had recommended but for a variety of reasons I never got around to it. The artane that he had prescribed changed the color of my urine to a bright yellow but did nothing for my Parkinson's. When the prescription for the artane ran out I did not get it refilled.

With the diagnosis finally complete it was time to learn something about...

9. The Disease

The disease was first defined in 1817 by the English physician James Parkinson, after whom the disease is named. He described it as "the shaking palsy." It has since been determined that Parkinson's disease is caused by a chemical imbalance in the brain. To be precise it is caused primarily by the loss of dopamine producing cells in an area of the brain known as the substantia nigra. Dopamine is the neurotransmitter that is manufactured in that part of the brain. It functions as the transmitter of nerve signals between the substantia nigra and the striatum. These nerve signals in turn control coordination and movement. When the supply of dopamine is reduced the signals are not properly transmitted, leading to coordination and movement problems in the afflicted person.

It has been estimated that there are approximately 400,000 dopamine-producing nerve cells in the substantia nigra, 200,000 on each side. It is believed that Parkinson's disease symptoms first appear when the disease has destroyed about 60 percent of the cells in the substantia nigra. When about 90 percent of the dopamine-producing nerve cells in the substantia nigra have been destroyed a person has advanced Parkinson's disease.

Parkinson's disease is best defined as a movement disorder. Its symptoms vary widely from one person to another. The wide range of variations found in the disease make treatment a very complicated issue. The most common symptom is an uncontrolled shaking or tremor that is found in about 75 percent of those afflicted. It is defined as a resting tremor that usually appears initially in one or both hands. As the disease progresses it usually spreads to other body parts, such as the arms and legs.

A person's walking ability or gait is frequently a very visible indication of Parkinson's disease. It is usually expressed by a slight hesitation in starting, slowness of movement and an overall lack of coordination. The natural swing of the arms is often impaired and is out of phase with the legs. Balance is impaired and changes in direction are sometimes difficult.

Bradykinesia is the clinical name for one of the more frustrating problems associated with Parkinson's disease. It is usually described as slowness of movement, and in extreme cases the inability to start a movement. When the beginning of a movement is delayed for several seconds, it is often referred to as "freezing." When freezing occurs the affected body part will not move until it gets the correct signal from the nervous system. Bradykinesia is often a major contributor to a lot of the problems encountered with walking and other movement activities.

Another symptom that is sometimes encountered with Parkinson's is a condition known as dyskinesia. It is defined as the involuntary movement of body parts, most commonly beginning with the hands and arms. It frequently occurs in people who are in the more advanced stages of the disease. While all of the symptoms of Parkinson's disease reduce the quality of life and are an embarrassment to the person afflicted, dyskinesia is considered by many to be the most cruel.

Rigidity or stiffness of movement is a common symptom of Parkinson's. It occurs in all body parts but is most often found in the arms and legs. It is caused by a reduction in the control of the counteracting muscles that would normally allow the smooth movement of body parts. For instance the arm is bent when the muscles that hold it straight relax and the muscles that bend the arm are tensed. When those muscles are not coordinated the arm movement is uneven and usually has a ratcheting appearance.

Other symptoms of Parkinson's disease are less obvious and are not unique to the disease. Stooped posture, sleep problems, small illegible handwriting, speech problems, constipation, drooling, problems with swallowing, and depression are sometimes encountered to various degrees.

For the most part my symptoms were similar to those of an average Parkinsonian. They first appeared in my early fifties, the usual age of those afflicted. Hand tremor was the first indication of trouble, followed by problems with running, and then with walking. By the time that I was finally diagnosed with Parkinson's I had accepted slowness of movement as a way of life. I had also experienced some problems with freezing, mostly with my left leg when attempting to start moving. Fortunately I have not yet encountered any problems with dyskinesia.

Having met and defined the disease it was now time to review my needs and responsibilities, examine my options and prepare...

PART FIVE

Into the Closet: Hiding Symptoms

10. The Game Plan

With the realization that I had a debilitating disease that was going to destroy my ability to earn a living, it seemed that I needed to establish my priorities. With three kids still in school it was more than obvious that I was going to have to stay employed as long as possible, because they would never get through college on my Social Security benefits. There was no guarantee that my present employer would be successful in the hazardous waste business, so I had to assume that I would once again join the ranks of the unemployed. I needed to answer the big question. Should I tell people that I had Parkinson's disease, or should I stay in the proverbial closet?

The employment situation in Houston had improved but there were still more engineers looking for work than the jobs that were available. I had to decide whether I could afford to place myself in a position where I would have to find an employer who would hire a person with Parkinson's disease, if a qualified healthy person were available. I felt that the answer to that question would nearly always be in the negative. I decided that I could not risk disclosing that I had Parkinson's. The day after the diagnosis I began a campaign to cover my Parkinson's symptoms. I had to hide my condition. Only my immediate family would know and they were to tell no one.

The only positive feature of my Parkinson's disease was that it had no impact on my thought processes or intellect. That situation meant that I could still do the work. The challenge, therefore, was to hide my physical defects. Prior to my cervical surgery I had explained to friends and co-workers that the calcium deposits inside my cervical vertebrae were distorting my spinal cord and were causing my tremor and coordination problems. To provide a believable cover for my Parkinson's I used the failed surgery ploy. The operation had been a success, but it had not been performed in a timely manner. I had sustained "permanent nerve damage." I told people that "things were not going to get any better, but fortunately, with a little luck they would not get much worse."

To hide my Parkinson's I felt that it was necessary to hide the symptoms of the disease as much as possible. My biggest fear was meeting someone who would recognize my Parkinson's symptoms. My challenge was to mask my symptoms to the point that my nerve damage story was believable.

The most obvious symptom that I needed to hide was my resting tremor, which at that time was most apparent in my hands. I never knew which hand would start shaking until it happened. To deal with that problem I discovered that the best cover was to grab something as quickly as possible. A piece of furniture would do nicely. The arm of a chair or the edge of a desktop became acceptable targets. If there was nothing solid to grab I would attack my body. Stuffing my hand into a pocket, hooking my thumb inside my belt, or grabbing an ear lobe became reasonably good distractions. If I was engaged in a conversation or at a meeting where the above distractions were not practical, I found that squeezing a pencil or a piece of paper sometimes helped lessen the tremor.

My next most obvious symptom was bradykinesia or slowness of movement. This problem was most apparent on occasions when I was starting a motion. It usually appeared as a hesitation when starting to walk or sometimes when getting out of a chair. If there were people nearby I would make a special effort to start fast. If things did not go smoothly I would fake a pained facial expression and grab my lower back with one or both hands. After a few weeks I was able to make a staggered start look a little like a chronic lower back problem.

The surgery that Dr. Cutler performed on my cervical vertebrae was, and is still, an item of considerable concern. Three and one half vertebrae at the back of my neck were no longer able to provide protection for my spinal cord. There was a gap of almost two inches where it was exposed to possible injury. A few months after the surgery I accidentally bumped the back of my neck while working in my garden. To say that it was an electrifying, eye-opening experience would be a reasonably accurate statement. I don't ever want to receive a real hit in that area.

The situation with my surgically weakened neck required a significant change in my lifestyle. I had to avoid any type of physical confrontation. A blow of any kind to my head could have a tragic result.

I had to avoid falling down, especially falling backwards. Falling backwards would probably cause the back of my head to contact the floor resulting in a serious head injury. To lessen the chance of an injury occurring in a fall I had to learn to walk with my weight slightly forward. In that posture, if I fell, I would fall forward and could use my hands to negotiate a soft landing.

Protecting my surgically weakened neck became a priority. I had to deal with the possibility that a whiplash injury could place me in a wheelchair for the rest of my life. To reduce the risk of that type of injury it was necessary for me to purchase a car that had a driver's seat with a good head restraint. The next thing that I did was to buy a head strap and add some neck exercises to my exercise program. I reasoned that if I kept my neck as strong as possible, it might enable me to avoid a serious injury in a minor accident.

My long-range retirement plans to play sixty plus ice hockey vanished with the backs of my cervical vertebrae. Ice hockey for old folks is a non-contact sport, but there are often collisions with players out of control. The possibility of an on-ice collision made that type of activity too risky.

Swallowing food became an item of considerable concern because inhaling food into the lungs could easily lead to pneumonia, which of course could be fatal. As a person who could talk and eat at the same time, I had to slow down and learn to swallow each mouthful very carefully.

Finally, but in no way less important, I had to use better judgment in dealing with medical practitioners. I was going to be a lot more involved in decisions about my treatment. If anything important arose I resolved to get at least two other opinions.

With the completion and implementation of the game plan it was time to make a comprehensive review of…

11. The Available Therapies

The Robin Williams movie "Awakenings" is all about the experimental drug L-dopa and its application by Dr. Malcolm Sayer to improve the lives of some of his catatonic patients. L-dopa was developed to treat Parkinson's disease by restoring some of the dopamine that has been lost to the disease. Better known today as levodopa, L-dopa is still the only drug that can deliver dopamine to the brain of a person with the disease. Levodopa therapy is universally accepted as the basic treatment for Parkinson's.

Levodopa therapy is not perfect because the drug does not easily penetrate the blood-brain barrier to enter the brain where it is converted into dopamine. When it was first used to treat Parkinson's disease overdosing quickly became a problem, because most physicians wanted to ensure that an acceptable quantity of levodopa reached the brain. Partly because of the overdosing long-term levodopa treatment was found to produce side effects that were unacceptable for most patients. Dyskinesia, the involuntary movement of body parts such as the arms and legs, was the primary problem in most cases.

It was eventually determined that the difficulty in penetrating the blood-brain barrier allowed most of the levodopa to be converted to dopamine in the blood before it could enter the brain. To reduce the side effects experienced with long-term levodopa treatment carbidopa was added as an inhibitor to block the conversion of levodopa to dopamine in the blood. With more of the levodopa in the dose now able to reach the brain, the quantity of levodopa in the dosage was drastically reduced. The reduced level of levodopa in the dosage made the drug much more predictable in its application and reduced the side effects. Levodopa, with carbidopa as an inhibitor, quickly became the drug of choice for the treatment of Parkinson's disease.

Symmetrel was initially developed as a flu prevention drug. In its application it was found that it reduced the tremor experienced by patients with Parkinson's disease. It is believed by some that symmetrel functions by releasing dopamine from the cells in the substantia nigra. That may or may not be correct. In any event it has been estimated that about half of the people who have taken symmetrel for Parkinson's have found it to be beneficial.

Deprenyl is the drug that was the primary focus of the DATATOP study in which I participated. It was developed in 1960 in Budapest and was first used in Europe as an anti-aging drug. In the middle of the nineteen-seventies the Europeans began using it to treat people with Parkinson's disease. When taken with levodopa it was found to be helpful in dealing with some of the movement problems associated with Parkinson's. The mechanism by which it achieved that result is unclear. It is believed by some that it retards the death of the cells of the substantia nigra. Deprenyl was not available in the United States when I was diagnosed with Parkinson's because it had not been approved by the Food and Drug Administration.

Another group of drugs described as dopamine agonists has been found to be helpful to some people with Parkinson's disease. These drugs are believed to mimic the action of dopamine in the brain by stimulating the dopamine receptors. Drugs that are available in this group include mirapex, requip, permax and parlodel. I have never used any of these drugs and cannot comment on their performance. They do however provide me with a viable "last resort" if or when my present regimen fails to control my Parkinson's.

Exercise therapy ranks right behind levodopa therapy as an effective treatment for people with Parkinson's disease. It is generally accepted that physical exercise stimulates the brain to produce dopamine. The quantity of dopamine produced varies widely with different individuals, as well as with the type and amount of exercise performed.

Exercise could be loosely defined as any activity that increases the heart rate. It can be further divided into exercises that for the most part work the skeletal muscles such as weight training, and those that primarily affect the cardiovascular system such as running. Exercises such as swimming and rowing work both the skeletal muscles and the cardiovascular system.

If a person has the wherewithal, physical therapy could be added to their treatment program. Physical therapy could be very helpful to people with Parkinson's disease if it enables them to participate in a worthwhile exercise program.

The list of available therapies for Parkinson's disease is far from impressive. Levodopa with carbidopa as an inhibitor is the only drug that is believed to actually replenish some of the dopamine in the brain that has been lost to the disease. Exercise is the only activity that is believed to result in the production of dopamine within the brain.

In short the treatment of Parkinson's disease boils down to exercise and levodopa or to put it more graphically, the dumb bells and dopamine of my title.

In 1987 some people with the disease who desperately wanted to be cured became the target of...

12. The Snake Oil Salesmen

They are as American as apple pie and baseball. The dictionary defines them as sellers of a "liquid cure-all with no medicinal value." The mixture usually had a significant alcohol content that sometimes compensated for its lack of curative value.

Snake oil salesmen first appeared around the middle of the nineteenth century, primarily in the Western States. Practitioners of that craft were usually silver-tongued rascals who were part of a traveling medicine show. They usually went from town to town hawking their worthless liquid as a cure for whatever ailed the people they met. With a little bit of luck they would be far away before their customers realized that they had been gulled. Occasionally a practitioner who failed to get far enough away was captured and subjected to another Americanism of the time, tar and feathers.

As the years passed patent medicines became available to cure most common ailments, and prescription drugs were developed to cure many diseases. To survive in the twentieth century the snake oil salesmen directed their attention to people who suffered from incurable afflictions or diseases. They concocted mixtures and procedures that were supposed to cure ailments that ranged from baldness to cancer. At the low end of the scale they functioned as sideshow barkers or door-to-door salesmen. At the top end they appeared as sophisticated practitioners operating out of well-organized medical clinics.

In 1987 Parkinsonians were bedeviled by conflicting reports of a cure for the disease that plagued them. A clinic in Mexico reported that it had obtained "distinct clinical improvement" from a surgical procedure performed on two patients with Parkinson's disease. The initial report was followed by another that the "improvement progressed rapidly." The news media in its endless lust for sensationalism, over-reacted to the positive aspects of that report. The New York Times, for instance, on April 2 of that year proclaimed that it was "the most dramatic development so far in the long, frustrating effort to treat Parkinson's disease." The news media continued to exploit the positive aspects of the event to the point that a lot of people were led to believe that Parkinson's disease had been cured. Unfortunately the unbridled press coverage was grossly inaccurate and led to an episode that could be referred to as "the great adrenal gland transplant scam."

Adrenal gland transplants were first attempted in Sweden in 1982, after it had been determined that a person's adrenal glands secreted a chemical similar to the dopamine that was produced in the substantia nigra. Transplant surgery had been performed on four patients with "very modest improvements." The surgical procedure had removed medullo-adrenal fragments from an adrenal gland of each patient and placed them in the striatum of the patient's brain. The objective of the procedure was to have the fragments bond with the striatum and produce an acceptable form of dopamine. The results were not encouraging and the project was abandoned.

The apparent success at the Mexican clinic was not consistent with the Swedish experience. An early comparison of results indicated that the Mexican patients were younger and that there were several differences in the surgical procedure. A detailed comparison of results was never attempted. People wanted to believe the positive aspects of the event and the glowing reports in the news media.

The impact of the Mexican report on people with Parkinson's disease was awesome. Everyone wanted to know more about the surgical procedure. A large number of people wanted to undergo the operation based on the results that had been obtained by the Mexican clinic on just two patients. What was even more amazing was that some people with Parkinson's disease actually went to medical facilities demanding that they be admitted for adrenal gland surgery.

The demand for this surgery at that time greatly exceeded the capacity of surgical facilities involved with neurological-transplants of any type. In a free society supply eventually equals demand. In this instance that basic law of economics held firm. In virtually no time at all the number of medical facilities performing adrenal gland transplants had increased to meet the demand. The ethics involved in the operation of some of those facilities, however, was much in question.

At that time I was not too interested in another surgery after my experience with Dr. Cutler. I was however very interested in a cure for Parkinson's disease. I read everything that I could find on adrenal gland transplants. It soon became apparent that not all of those in the medical community were convinced that the much-desired cure had been found. Some neurologists were trying to bring some sanity to the situation. They were concerned that the expectations were too high, based on just two apparently successful procedures. They were advising caution. My own neurologist was very skeptical and wanted to see a lot more data.

In spite of the lack of confirmation as to its success adrenal gland transplants continued. For many people the prospect of being cured far outweighed the risks involved. The demand for transplants was so strong at that time that the standing joke in the medical community concerned the absence of animal testing of the procedure. The tongue-in-cheek response was that the procedure was considered unsafe for animals so they were using humans.

In 1988 the International Parkinson's Disease Conference in Jerusalem reported on about fifty adrenal transplants that had been performed worldwide. The report was considered to be very negative as only about a third of the patients showed any improvement and there had been several deaths. At that point in time common sense alone should have resulted in a halt to adrenal transplants. Professional ethics in the medical community should have led to the same conclusion. However neither prevailed.

Postmortems on people who had died following adrenal gland transplant surgery showed that the implanted fragments were "completely atrophied and sclerotic and incapable of exercising the dopaminergic effect on the striatum." In plain language the fragments had not taken root, had dried out and died. That determination and the knowledge that the adrenal gland secretion was only similar to, not the same as, the dopamine in the substantia nigra, should have ended the transplant mania.

Unfortunately the snake oil practitioners had obtained a solid footing. Demand for the procedure was still strong and they were experiencing occasional short-term success with some patients. Their clinics were making money and they were not about to terminate the golden goose. It seemed that as long as there was somebody with the prescribed amount of money, who was willing to undergo the procedure, there would be a clinic that was willing to provide the service.

It has been estimated that about three hundred adrenal gland transplants were performed worldwide before the demand abated. It has also been estimated that less than 20 percent of the patients received any benefit from the surgery. The number of patients who received any real benefit is unknown. The number of deaths directly related to the surgery is also unknown.

A great deal of money had been scammed and a lot of people had been damaged. There is no record that anybody was ever arrested or charged with criminal intent. The experimental nature of the surgery probably provided an acceptable legal loophole for those involved. There is also no record that anybody was tarred and feathered, although some practitioners surely deserved that treatment.

After accepting the fact that I had an incurable disease it was time to move on. It was time to make a decision about my participation in…

PART SIX

The Deprenyl Story: Bureaucratic Bungling

13. The DATATOP Study

The DATATOP study was a multi-center, multi-million dollar investigation sponsored by the Parkinson Study Group in Rochester, New York. Its name was derived from its title, the Deprenyl And Tocopherol Anti-oxidative Therapy Of Parkinsonism. The study was conducted at twenty-two centers throughout the United States and Canada.

To set the scene at the start of the study it is necessary to know that deprenyl and tocopherol are classified as anti-oxidation drugs. Tocopherol is a non-prescription drug better known as vitamin E. Deprenyl is the drug that was developed in Budapest in 1960 as an anti-aging drug, and had been used in Europe to treat Parkinson's disease since the middle of the nineteen-seventies. At the time of the study deprenyl did not have approval for use in either the United States or Canada.

The purpose of the study was to examine the safety and effectiveness of deprenyl and tocopherol on people in the early stages of Parkinson's disease. The study was designed specifically to determine if the application of those drugs would slow the progression of the disease. The goal was to determine if the drugs could extend the period of time before levodopa therapy became necessary.

The candidates for the study were subjected to the usual blarney that their contribution may "bring a brighter future for you and other patients with Parkinson's disease." I did not believe that they could learn very much from either vitamin E or a drug that had been in use in Europe for more than ten years. In spite of my doubts about the value of the study I decided to participate. My decision was not based on any noble thoughts about my contribution to medical science. It was based on the expectation that through interaction with other participants and the medical professionals who ran the study I would learn more about the disease. Since I did not expect that I would ever have enough time to locate or read the books recommended by Dr. Knowles I hoped that DATATOP would fill some of that gap.

Candidates for the study were people who had recently been diagnosed with Parkinson's disease. The most important requirement was that the candidates had never been exposed to levodopa therapy. In fact they preferred that the candidates be free of any drug therapy. Age and gender were unimportant, however they tried to have an equal number of men and women.

At 9:30 on the morning of November 30, 1987, my fifty-fifth birthday, I began my participation in the DATATOP study. After completing the required paperwork and providing blood and urine samples I was subjected to a baseline clinical examination. That examination was designed primarily to provide a comprehensive assessment of my motor functions. The tests ranged from simple movements such as touching thumb to forefinger, drawing freehand circles and rising from a chair. I believe that I was able to perform all of the movements, but some of them were done rather slowly.

In the afternoon I checked into the hospital for the piece de resistance, a spinal tap. I do not remember how they talked me into that test because it was just about as much fun as Dr. Cutler's myelograph. For reasons unknown they needed a sample of my cerebrospinal fluid and inserting a needle into my spinal cord was supposed to be the easiest way to get it.

The participants in the study were assigned to one of four groups. Each group consisted of the same number of people, with people of about the same age and gender in each of the four groups. The project was conducted as a double blind study. That meant that neither the participants, nor the study administrators, knew to which group a person had been assigned. In my case it could have been considered a triple blind because I was never able to meet or interact with any of the other people who participated in the study. The net result was that I got less out of the study than I had expected.

To determine the effectiveness of deprenyl and tocopherol the study designers chose to add a non-drug, i.e. a placebo, to the mix. Each of the four groups was assigned a different combination of medications. One group received deprenyl and tocopherol. Another group got deprenyl and the third group received tocopherol. The final group got a dose of nothing, the placebo treatment.

The following tabulation lists the specifics of the medication that was provided to each group.

Deprenyl/tocopherol group.

> 5 mg deprenyl tablet twice daily.
> 1000 I.U. tocopherol capsule twice daily.

Deprenyl group.

> 5 mg deprenyl tablet twice daily.
> Inactive capsule identical to tocopherol twice daily.

Tocopherol group.

> 1000 I.U. tocopherol capsule twice daily.
> Inactive tablet identical to deprenyl twice daily.

Placebo group.

> Inactive tablet identical to deprenyl twice daily.
> Inactive capsule identical to tocopherol twice daily.

The placebo group was an important addition to the study because it was possible that neither deprenyl, nor tocopherol, would be effective in delaying the advance of Parkinson's disease. The placebo group was used as a point of reference to measure the effectiveness of the medications on the other groups. With three of the four groups receiving an active drug, the probability that I would avoid the placebo group seemed very good.

At the completion of the baseline evaluation I began the drug therapy provided by the DATATOP study group. My first impression of the medication was a small increase in my energy level. That pretty well convinced me that I had avoided the dreaded placebo group and was receiving one of the active medications. As the months passed there did not seem to be any significant decrease in the rate at which my Parkinsonism advanced. I decided to stay with the program because the rate of my decline seemed to be acceptable.

I returned to the study center for follow-up evaluations at one month, three months and six months after starting the study. I decided to withdraw from the study before my ninth month evaluation. My decision to withdraw from the study became necessary when my employer decided to withdraw from the hazardous waste business. They decided to make a clean sweep of things and fired the entire design group. Once more I was on the outside looking in. I was going to need all the help I could get to retard the advance of my Parkinson's disease. I needed to start levodopa therapy.

For my part I had my final evaluation in September of 1988, an event that included providing blood and urine samples. It also included another spinal tap that was just about as much fun as the baseline event.

They continued the DATATOP study to the end of 1992 with the involvement of about a thousand participants. In January of 1993 I received a letter from the Parkinson Study Group which informed me that I had received both deprenyl and tocopherol during the clinical phase of the study. It also stated that I was "part of the largest, longest-running study on the treatment of patients with early, untreated Parkinson's disease."

The letter went on to state that I had "helped to advance knowledge about this disease and its treatments." It was written and signed by the two gentlemen who were in charge of the study. I was considering having it framed until I took a closer look at the signatures and realized that their secretaries had signed the letter.

The results of the DATATOP study showed that most participants who received deprenyl experienced a longer time period before levodopa treatment was required. The study did not quantify the time period that could be expected before levodopa therapy would be needed. It also showed that tocopherol was not effective in delaying the progression of Parkinson's disease. I had expected more from a study that took almost five years and cost millions of dollars to complete.

Over the years I was to learn that a great deal of time and money used for Parkinson's research was spent on studies like DATATOP, instead of looking for a cure. A lot of people work very hard to raise money for Parkinson's disease research and a lot of that money is wasted on projects that seem to be designed to bring a degree of notoriety to a few individuals with little if any benefit to people with the disease. The DATATOP study could be considered as a classic example of how to waste both time and money.

My involvement with deprenyl research ended with my departure from the DATATOP study. However no discussion of deprenyl could be complete without acknowledging the contribution made by...

14. The Family Dog

This episode in the history of deprenyl was mostly due to the efforts of a very colorful individual who lived north of the border. Dr. Morton Shulman was a medical doctor who became very well known for the outrageous actions that he directed at the Canadian political system. The ruling party in the Province of Ontario was one of his frequent targets. One of his favorite tricks was to photograph cabinet ministers sleeping while the house was in session. All politicians strive to be on camera as much as possible, but not on the six o'clock news when they are asleep on the job.

In the summer of 1981 he was literally in hog heaven. In addition to his medical practice he hosted a weekly television show and was writing a newspaper column, both of which were confrontational and stirred the pot. Life was good. In fact it was so good that it could only go downhill, and downhill it went.

Things began to come unglued when he noticed a slight tremor in his left leg. In a matter of weeks it had developed into a noticeable shuffle when he walked. His condition went from bad to worse and by September of that year he was diagnosed as a certifiable member of the Parkinson's community.

He began levodopa therapy and things returned to normal, but at a much slower pace. His life was acceptable until the spring of 1987 when his body virtually crashed. He had great difficulty in starting any type of movement. His tremor had also returned. He needed help in getting out of bed, and also needed a cane when walking around the house. A friend told him about a drug that was used in Europe for the treatment of Parkinson's disease. The drug was named deprenyl and it had been used with some degree of success for a number of years.

Another friend who was visiting in Europe was able to obtain one hundred tablets of deprenyl for his use. When he added deprenyl to his levodopa therapy his tremor was reduced and his mobility improved. His energy level also increased and he justifiably viewed deprenyl as something just short of a miracle. When he realized that he had stumbled onto a pill that he could buy for a dime and sell for a buck he probably also viewed it as some sort of gold mine.

In August of 1987 he acquired the right to market deprenyl in Canada from an American company. While he had the right to market the drug in Canada, he did not have the approval of Canada's Department of Health and Welfare. Deprenyl had not been approved for use in Canada because nobody had ever applied for its approval. Starting at square one to obtain Canadian approval would probably take years.

He decided to take his battle for deprenyl approval south of the border where the Food and Drug Administration (FDA) was close to approving its use in the United States. An application for approval of deprenyl for the treatment of Parkinson's disease had been filed with the FDA several years before. It had not been approved because the FDA was unwilling to accept some of the test data submitted by the European companies. The bone of contention seemed to be the lack of a suitable toxicology test report. The FDA apparently required a toxicity test where deprenyl would be fed to rats for a period of one year. The European test period was six months. The fact that humans had been taking it for years in Europe without a single toxic incident was of no consequence. The FDA still wanted their rat test.

To break the impasse Dr. Shulman needed some way to pressure the FDA into accepting the European test data. Once again he concocted an outrageous solution. He announced that he was going to seek approval to use deprenyl as an additive to dog food. Knowing that deprenyl was created as an anti-aging drug he argued that dog owners would gladly pay for a drug that could possibly extend the life of a faithful pet. The family dog was about to spearhead the battle for the approval of deprenyl.

To say that the FDA was not amused by his proposal was perhaps the understatement of the year. They were probably terrified. The FDA had been placed in the position where they faced the ridiculous prospect of a large number of people with Parkinson's disease acquiring a real or an imaginary family dog, and buying deprenyl from a friendly neighborhood veterinarian. There was an immediate reaction from various government agencies on both sides of the border regarding the possibility that a veterinarian could be permitted to dispense a prescription drug for dogs that would be used by people with Parkinson's disease.

There is no evidence that the family dog ploy had any influence on the FDA's decision regarding deprenyl. It is, however, a fact that in June of 1989, a few months after the above incident, the FDA announced that it had approved the use of deprenyl for the treatment of Parkinson's disease.

A few days after my final evaluation for the DATATOP study I was ready to begin levodopa therapy. It seemed like a good time to review the available therapies and begin…

PART SEVEN

The Never Ending Story: Living with Parkinson's Disease

15. The Selected Treatment

It has been established that levodopa is the only medication that can replenish some of the dopamine in the substantia nigra that has been lost to the disease. Exercise is believed to be the only activity that can actually cause the nerve cells in the substantia nigra to produce a little more dopamine. That was the situation when I was diagnosed with Parkinson's disease almost twenty years ago and that is still the situation today.

With the knowledge that all of the drugs used to treat Parkinson's disease lose their effectiveness over time it was obvious that the most important therapy in the treatment of my Parkinson's disease was going to be a well managed drug program. A successful program would have to be keyed to get the maximum benefit from levodopa therapy.

It has also been established that the length of time that a drug is effective depends in part on its rate of use, or to be specific, its dosage. A drug taken at a low dosage would therefore be expected to be effective for a longer period of time than if it were taken at a high dosage. The selected therapy would therefore consist of the careful selection of supporting medications and a rigorous exercise program to minimize the use of levodopa.

I began levodopa therapy in 1988 after leaving the DATATOP study. I started with carbidopa/levodopa and symmetrel. Symmetrel was selected to support my levodopa therapy because it helps in controlling tremor, which was, and is still the biggest problem created by my Parkinson's disease. My drug regimen at that time consisted of:

1- 25/100 mg carbidopa/levodopa tablet 3 times a day
1- 100 mg symmetrel capsule 2 times a day

I began levodopa therapy with some trepidation because I was well aware that about 30 percent of the people with Parkinson's do not respond positively to that medication. If I did not respond positively to that very important drug I was going to have real problems with Parkinson's disease.

I can still remember taking that first carbidopa/levodopa tablet and waiting for a reaction. About half an hour after taking that tablet I began to experience a positive reaction. After a few more minutes I was able to move and function like a normal person. It seemed like some sort of miracle. After about an hour the levodopa induced boost started to wear off and things began to slow down. However things never got all the way back to the unmedicated condition. About six hours after I took the first tablet I took another and the on-off process was repeated.

My initial drug regimen could be considered as the typical beginner's therapy for a person with Parkinson's disease. I felt that the medication gave me more of a boost than I needed and I thought that the levodopa dosage could be reduced. However the selected drugs were doing a very good job of masking my Parkinson's so I decided not to consider making any changes at that time. I did not want to rock the boat.

Over the years I was to learn that the on-off cycle for levodopa therapy usually varied a little from day to day. For reasons unknown the time required to kick in sometimes increased to hours instead of minutes and the boost was less than normal. I have never been able to accurately predict when the on-cycle would begin. However if I was in a stressful situation I could expect the on-cycle to be delayed and the boost to be reduced. That was not the best arrangement because it was difficult to control my tremor when the levodopa was not working properly. A stressful situation could be caused by something as simple as having to explain why I was delayed in completing an assignment. It became just one more thing that I had to be aware of, and learn to live with.

I discovered soon after starting levodopa therapy that if I got into a very stressful situation, such as an argument with someone, my Parkinson's disease would sometimes break through the medication. When a breakthrough occurred I would virtually come unglued. My symptoms would be a lot worse than what I would expect to encounter in an unmedicated condition. My hands and arms would shake uncontrollably and I would be unable to speak coherently. I would be unable to frame as much as a simple sentence. A confrontation of that type had to be avoided. It had to become an absolute no-no. That was not a good situation to have to live with in the work-a-day world.

Deprenyl was added to my regimen to support the levodopa therapy when it became available in June of 1989. At that time my Parkinson's medication consisted of:

1- 25/100 mg carbidopa/levodopa tablet 3 times a day.
1- 100 mg symmetrel capsule 2 times a day.
1- 5 mg deprenyl tablet 2 times a day.

It appears that I have been one of the lucky ones because my response to all of my Parkinson's drugs has been better than good. Whenever possible all medications were taken on an empty stomach at least a half-hour before eating. This was done to allow maximum absorption through the digestive system into the blood. Medications were also taken at the same time each day so that the body would become accustomed to processing the various chemicals contained in the drugs. The times when medications were taken were selected so that the interval between doses was about the same and a relatively constant level of the drug was maintained in the bloodstream. If a medication was not taken at its scheduled time because of an oversight, the medication would not be doubled when the next dose was taken.

Side effects to my medications have been minimal to date and the only significant problem was sleep related. After beginning levodopa therapy there was a minor problem with hallucinations that caused me to imagine small animals, usually cats or dogs, racing around my bedroom. The only significant event that occurred during that period happened one night during an unusually vivid display when I decided to participate. I tried to swat one of the critters when it came into range. Unfortunately my roundhouse right nailed the lamp on my bedside table. With the loss of a perfectly good reading lamp I decided that in the future I would remain a spectator instead of trying to become a participant. Over time the episodes became less frequent and less vivid. After about a year the hallucinations were down to about one episode a month and no longer a problem.

Generic substitutes are available for each of the three drugs in my daily regimen and I have used generics for all three of my drugs. I have found that some of the generic products have produced inconsistent results. Some medications seemed to have too much strength, others not enough. At first I thought it was caused by a good day, bad day syndrome on my part.

A review of the situation disclosed that the chemical composition of brand name drugs can vary plus or minus 10% from standard. Generics are permitted to vary plus or minus 20% from standard. That equated to a 40% swing between high and low, a range that appeared to be unacceptable. I eventually discovered that the wide variation for the most part was between the different manufacturers of generics. If I stayed with the same manufacturer things seemed to remain on target.

To reduce the range between high and low response to levodopa medication, a controlled release or CR product has been developed and is widely used in the treatment of Parkinson's. I have used that medication and found it to be unsuitable with my low dosage regimen. With the CR product I could never tell when or if the drug kicked in. In the final analysis I felt that the level of levodopa absorption into my bloodstream had been reduced by using the CR product and my activity level had suffered. After a three-month trial I switched back to the regular product.

To learn that exercise was an important therapy for people with Parkinson's disease was something like winning the Florida State Lottery on a single ticket. Many years ago I decided that I was going to pursue a very active lifestyle. To achieve that goal it was necessary for me to maintain a relatively high level of physical fitness. A friend of mine introduced me to weight training with barbells and dumb bells during my first year of college. It was virtually a case of love at first sight. Weight training, a form of progressive resistance exercise, became the keystone in my quest for physical fitness and an activity that I practiced on a regular basis for virtually all of my adult life. I was fortunate to have a dedicated exercise program in place when Parkinson's arrived, because that activity was to become a major factor in controlling the advance of the disease.

I began weight training in September of 1951 at the age of 18. At that time Arnold Schwarzenegger was just 4 years old. Facilities for weight training in 1951 were virtually non-existent because coaches and trainers in those days believed that people who participated in that activity would become muscle-bound. I was never able to determine exactly what the condition entailed, because I was never able to find anybody who suffered from that affliction. In 1951 if you wanted to work out with weights you probably had to join your neighborhood YMCA. If you did not have a YMCA in your neighborhood, and you wanted to train with weights you were forced to improvise.

I began with a plate-loaded barbell and two plate-loaded dumb bells that I had purchased from a mail-order catalogue. There was no room in our basement so I began my quest for physical fitness by lifting weights in my bedroom. I was able to cobble together a bench with brackets to hold the barbell for bench presses, an incline board for abdominal exercises and a crude squat rack. It did not look like much, but it was enough to provide the basic facilities for weight training. I worked out three days a week, every week, and was able to make respectable gains in strength and muscle size over the next two years. Lifting weights in my bedroom was the beginning of my lifelong involvement with weight training.

In 1966 at the age of 34, I decided to add some cardio-vascular work to my exercise routine. I began running and in about two months I was able to cover two miles without stopping, in a respectable time. My exercise routine has been virtually unchanged since that date. I ran three days a week and three days a week I trained with weights. I ran two miles each workout until around 1990 when I reduced the distance to about a mile.

My weight training routines however have varied over the years to suit the equipment that was available in the places where I worked out. I always preferred to use barbells and dumb bells because you have to control the weight when you exercise and that in turn works a lot of minor muscles that are often by-passed when you use machines. Barbells and dumb bells are usually referred to as free weights, and I still believe that they provide the best type of resistance exercise.

I have used most of the exercise machines that are available today and have found that most of them are a very good form of resistance exercise. This is especially true of the machines that are designed to exercise a specific muscle, or group of muscles, by using pulleys or levers to life a stack of plates. It should also be noted that some of the exercise machines advertised on television seem to have been designed more for profit than fitness.

An average workout today usually consists of about fifteen exercises that take about forty-five minutes to complete. I always start with leg exercises, followed by arms, chest, shoulders, upper back and abdominals. The weights used in the various exercises have decreased considerably over the years, while my time to run a given distance has naturally increased.

I have found that exercise is not just important for people with Parkinson's disease. It is essential. In my case it is the glue that holds my low dosage medication regimen together. The truth of that statement has been demonstrated at times when I left home to visit family or friends and was unable to work out with weights, or run.

Without some type of rigorous exercise I would experience a minor meltdown after two or three days. My tremor would increase to the point where I had trouble functioning. It would be a struggle to use a knife and fork when eating. Drinking soup was impossible. Things would return to normal a few days after returning home and getting back into my exercise routine.

There are many reasons why a person should participate in a well-planned exercise routine that works both the skeletal muscles and the cardio-vascular system. Control of Parkinson's disease however does not seem to need that level of dedication. I have found that virtually any type of exercise will benefit a person with Parkinson's to some degree.

There have been times when I was away from home, and unable to work out with weights, I found that if I ran every day I was able to avoid most of the problems associated with the disease. It seemed that if I was able to run enough to break a sweat, and was able to hold it for about ten to fifteen minutes, the Parkinson's exercise demand for that day would be satisfied.

The type of exercise program selected for an individual with Parkinson's depends mostly on the physical condition of that individual. I believe that the best type of exercise for any individual is some form of resistance exercise, and the best type of resistance exercise is weight training. The amount of exercise a person should have is not an easy question to answer. A question that can be answered with some degree of accuracy would be how much exercise is too much. In that case there is a workable yardstick. That yardstick is the level of pain experienced during or after an exercise session. The only pain that a person should accept without question is a low level muscle pain. Events such as joint pain, chest pain and breathing problems should not be accepted without professional guidance.

Physical fitness equipment and facilities have made huge advances since 1951. There is no reason why any person with Parkinson's today would be unable to develop a beneficial exercise program. Just about every neighborhood has a fitness center that could design a suitable routine for anyone with the disease. For the stay-at-homes there is a wide range of equipment that can be purchased at a local discount store. A person with the disease simply has to decide to take charge of his or her life, begin an exercise program, and just do it.

Over the years I have been somewhat amazed at the low regard that most of the books on Parkinson's disease have for the value of exercise in the treatment of the disease. If it is mentioned at all, it is usually defined by a very low impact program that is virtually useless. To compound the problem, a lot of those programs are structured for just one day a week. Anything less than three days a week would probably be useless. The intensity level, even at low impact, should enable the person to break a sweat.

Exercising should always be done at least an hour after eating, because it is unwise to engage in physical activity while the body is digesting food. In my early years with the disease, when I was working I exercised just before dinner and would experience a significant, if temporary, boost in my energy level and coordination. Since retiring I usually work out before breakfast and even though the exercise-induced boost is much reduced it is still there.

It may not be correct to classify a person's diet as a therapy. However I have found that it is important to maintain what is usually considered to be a healthy diet. I usually eat low protein meals that include lots of fresh fruits and vegetables. I also try to include foods that are high in fiber, low in salt and saturated fat.

There are two significant conflicts between diet and drug therapy. Firstly, protein will consume some of the levodopa in carbidopa/levodopa and will reduce the effectiveness of that very important medication. If a protein rich meal is planned the medication should be taken at least an hour before eating. Secondly, if you are taking deprenyl, it is recommended that wine and cheese be avoided.

With a basic understanding of the disease and a treatment plan in place I thought that my life would return to some semblance of normalcy. That was not to be the case. The social system in which we live was to deliver two more major disruptions. The first one came from…

16. The Insurance Industry

To provide coverage at a reasonable rate an insurance company sometimes excludes a pre-existing condition from its policy. The insured person accepts responsibility for the excluded item and purchases a policy that provides coverage for the items not excluded. In that manner the insured deals with the known condition and buys coverage for the unknown.

The Consolidated Omnibus Budget Reconciliation Act of 1986 or COBRA as it is known, provides for health benefits after employment. When I became unemployed in 1988 I was able to continue my health insurance under COBRA by continuing to pay my employee portion of the monthly premium. I believe that arrangement lasted about a year. I then had the option of continuing the coverage for a longer period by adding the employer contribution to my monthly premium payment. After reviewing the coverage with the increased premium I felt I could get by with less coverage at a lower cost at another insurance company. On the assumption that my Parkinson's disease would be excluded from my next insurance coverage as a pre-existing condition I allowed my COBRA backed insurance to expire.

Shortly after my insurance coverage expired I made an application to a national insurance carrier for health insurance. About two weeks after making the application my check was returned, insurance denied, no reason given. An application to two other insurance companies produced the same result. That was not the response that I had expected. It was however another example of how easily things can go terribly wrong when you are battling a debilitating disease.

Fearing the worst I called a Parkinson's hot line provided by one of the national Parkinson's associations. The person who answered confirmed that insurance companies will not sell health insurance to people with Parkinson's disease. It seemed that I had painted myself into a corner. I was in a situation where I had no options and would have to wait until I was retired and could qualify for Medicare health insurance. In the interim I would have to do my very best to avoid a serious injury or illness.

A few months after the health insurance disaster I received my automobile insurance renewal notice. In an attempt to save a buck I applied to another company for a quotation. I was not required to disclose that I had Parkinson's disease and I did not make that disclosure. The result was the same as it was with the health insurance companies. Insurance denied, no reason given.

The denial of automobile insurance confirmed that I had been blackballed by the insurance industry because of my Parkinson's disease. I renewed my automobile insurance with my existing carrier expecting that I would be stuck with that carrier for the rest of my life. In retrospect I should have been more vigilant regarding my health insurance. On the other hand it would have been very helpful if just one of those Parkinson's disease booklets had explained the facts of life regarding the insurance industry.

With my Parkinson's disease symptoms becoming difficult to conceal, my employability becoming questionable, it was time to take note of the handwriting on the wall. It was time to accept the inevitable and prepare for…

PART EIGHT

Out of the Closet: Retirement

17. The Last Hurrah

With the demise of our design group in 1988 I again found myself among the unemployed. My situation however was considerably different from what it had been when I was unemployed in 1983. At that time there were no prospects of employment. This time the hazardous waste business was very strong and I knew some of the players.

I could have obtained employment at one of the companies in the hazardous waste business where I knew some people. However, realizing that I had only a few years of employability left, I decided to work as a consultant which would pay a little more if I could stay busy. I gambled that the hazardous waste business would remain strong until Parkinson's disease made me unemployable.

That decision proved to be a good choice as I was able to stay busy until early 1993, when I again found myself completely out of work without any prospects. At that time my Parkinson's disease had advanced to the point where my tremor could no longer be masked. It had also destroyed my handwriting to the point where it was barely legible. My brain could still do the work, but my body could no longer deliver the finished product. There was no way that I could disguise or hide my tremor during a job interview. I would have to tell the interviewer that I had Parkinson's disease. My chances of finding a job were just about zero.

It was time to bring down the curtain. My engineering career, that had lasted almost thirty-eight years, had ended, not with a bang, but with a whimper. When I began working in 1955 I never expected to do great things or to be anything other than a good engineer. I did not expect that I would spend over three years in a situation where I would be unable to find a real job. I surely never expected it to end when I was sixty years old, unemployable, with a debilitating disease. It seems that life is seldom what you expect it to be.

My engineering career had ended. Two of my three kids had completed college. The third was in his final year. There was no reason to remain in Houston. It was time to make…

18. The Big Move

The Gulf Coast region of southeast Texas, with its multiplicity of chemical plants and refineries, is considered by many to be the cancer capital of the world. From my observations of the number of people in attendance at some of the Parkinson's symposiums that I attended while living in Houston it could also be the Parkinson's disease capital. I will never know how I acquired Parkinson's disease, but living in Houston ranks high on my list of probable causes.

The first order of business at the beginning of my retirement was to get out of Houston. The second thing was to find a location where I could expect to spend the rest of my days. My first priority was a location below the snow line. The second was to be on or near a beach, where the air was clean and the water unpolluted. California faded from the scene when I saw that beach area property prices were way beyond my means. The second choice was the sunshine state, Florida. With the knowledge that most of the hurricanes came ashore on the Atlantic side I decided to relocate to the Gulf Coast.

In the spring of 1993 I rented an apartment on the Gulf Coast and began looking for a permanent home. After a lot of legwork I purchased a somewhat neglected edifice, near a white sand beach, on a barrier island.

The second order of business was to find a competent neurologist. The Parkinson's hot line gave me the names of several in my immediate area. My first selection was a young woman who assured me that my Parkinson's symptoms could easily be diagnosed as essential tremor. I assumed that she made that statement in defense of Dr. Timmons' incorrect diagnosis. While it may have been an impressive display of female solidarity it was not what I wanted to hear from a person who was going to be my neurologist.

My second selection was a young man who began our first meeting by making a basic neurological examination complete with rubber hammer and tuning fork. At the conclusion of his examination he confirmed that I had Parkinson's disease. Needless to say I was somewhat relieved to hear that I had not wasted the last five years treating the wrong affliction. He had some sales literature on his desk for a new drug that had recently been approved for the treatment of Parkinson's disease. Without assessing my present medication regimen he asked if I would like to try the latest FDA approved product. I considered his cavalier approach to my medication regimen to be unacceptable and decided to look elsewhere for a neurologist.

With two misfires in my search for a neurologist, I decided to step back and review the situation. I had been on the same medication for about five years without any problems. I had no intention of changing the medication as long as it controlled the disease at an acceptable level. I decided that I did not really need a neurologist. What I needed was an old fashioned general practitioner.

There was a small clinic on the island that specialized in family care. The members of the clinic were board certified in family medicine. I assumed that those people were the upgraded, modern day version of general practitioners. An appointment with Dr. Gloria Hunter confirmed that I would not need a neurologist to continue an established and successful treatment regimen. Dr. Hunter advised me that if my Parkinson's got out of control she would not be able to prescribe a change in my medication. In that event I would have to see a neurologist. That sounded like an ideal arrangement. My search for a competent physician had ended.

At that time it became painfully apparent to me that I should have obtained the services of a family medicine practitioner way back when I began having problems. I feel quite certain that if I had made that choice, I would have been dealing with an individual who would have known that cervical spondylosis had nothing to do with Parkinson's disease. The fiasco generated by those self-serving specialists, which led to an unnecessary surgery, would never have happened. I would not have had a cervical laminectomy. I probably would have played sixty plus ice hockey and I would have enjoyed a better quality of life.

In the spring of 1994, after I had settled into life in the slow lane, I decided to revisit the dosage of the medications that I was taking. I noticed that the boost generated by my drug regimen was often too high. At the start of the boost I was able to move very quickly and felt as if I had enough energy to climb a wall. At the other end of the spectrum when the boost abated, my energy level dropped so fast that my legs virtually buckled. The energy swing from high to low seemed to be excessive, and was an indication that I was probably over medicating.

To get things back on track I reduced the carbidopa/levodopa in my daily regimen to two tablets per day. To smooth out the digestion process I broke the tablets in half and took a half tablet four times a day. The net result was that my boost leveled out, my tremor was a little more obvious, but could still be managed.

The change meant that I had reduced my carbidopa/levodopa consumption by thirty-three percent. That could equate to a thirty-three percent extension in the length of time that it would be effective in controlling my Parkinson's disease. The possibility of a thirty-three percent extension in my useful life was a huge bonus. I felt that most of that bonus was probably due to my retirement from the stresses of the work-a-day world, and my move away from the Houston area and its industrial pollution.

A few weeks after the carbidopa/levodopa change had leveled out, I tried to reduce the symmetrel dosage. I cut it back to one per day and found that my tremor increased to an unmanageable level in about three days. I returned to two per day and the tremor was back to normal in about two days. That adjustment to my medication obviously did not work. The failed attempt to reduce my symmetrel dosage confirmed that the correct dosage for me at that time was two per day. In the unexpected bonus department, I have not had the flu since I began taking symmetrel. My self-adjusted drug regimen was now:

½ - 25/100 mg carbidopa/levodopa tablet 4 times a day
1 - 100 mg symmetrel capsule 2 times a day
1 - 5 mg deprenyl tablet 2 times a day

In the winter of 1996 I discovered that virtually all of the people in my support group who were taking deprenyl were taking one tablet per day. Most of them had their dosage reduced from two tablets per day, to one per day, to improve their sleep process. I reduced my deprenyl dosage to one per day to determine if the reduction would have any impact on the level of my Parkinson's symptoms. The change made a small improvement in my ability to get a good night's sleep with no significant change in the control of my Parkinson's disease. I decided to stay with the lower dosage of the deprenyl. There have been no changes since that date and my drug regimen today remains at:

½ - 25/100 mg carbidopa/levodopa tablet 4 times a day
1 - 100 mg symmetrel capsule 2 times a day
1 - 5 mg deprenyl tablet 1 time a day

This is a low dosage drug regimen by any standard and I feel fortunate to be able to function effectively with it. The only explanation that I have as to why it works for me probably rests with my long dedication to weight training and running. My diet may also be a contributing factor because I always try to eat what are generally considered to be healthy foods. A positive attitude, born out of the stubborn streak that I inherited from my father, has probably also been a factor in dealing with the disease.

In the spring of 1993, a few weeks after arriving in Florida, I was able to direct my attention to the problem created by what I have previously described as the second major disruption. I began what turned out to be a long-drawn-out battle with…

19. The Social Security Administration

The Social Security Administration was established on August 14, 1935 when President Franklin D. Roosevelt signed the Social Security Act into law. It was designed to pay retired workers, sixty-five years of age and older, a continuing income after retirement. On August 1, 1956 disability benefits were added for workers fifty years of age and older. Health benefits were added when President Lyndon B. Johnson initiated Medicare on July 30, 1965.

In the spring of 1993 after arriving in Florida I applied for disability benefits from the Social Security Administration. On July 1, 1993 I received a form letter stating that I was "not entitled to disability benefits." I could hardly believe my eyes. I had expended a lot of time and effort over the last five years looking for ways to stay employed instead of throwing in the towel and seeking disability benefits. I did not want to abuse the system, as so many people appear to have done. I believed that I had worked as long as I could and now the Social Security Administration was telling me that I did not qualify for benefits.

Again it would have been nice if just one of those booklets on Parkinson's disease had alerted me about the situation with Social Security. As it was with the Insurance Industry, there was no mention of the issues related to Social Security benefits and once more I had been blindsided by the system.

The letter went on to say that my "medical record" showed that I may "no longer be capable of performing work" that I had "performed in the past." It also stated that based on my "age, education, and past work experience," I was still "capable of performing other work which requires less physical effort."

"Other work which requires less physical effort." I was a design engineer. I sat at a desk, made calculations, wrote specifications and performed other non-physical tasks. In spite of my best efforts I was never able to find employment that required less physical effort than lifting a pencil or operating a calculator.

The letter closed with information on how I was to proceed with my appeal. It stated that my local Social Security office had "a list of groups" that could help with my appeal. It also informed me that there were lawyers who did not charge for their services unless I won my appeal. The letter stated that if I hired someone, the Social Security Administration "must approve the fee before he or she can collect it." It seemed that the Social Security Administration expected people to appeal their unfavorable decisions. They had established exactly how an appeal was to be presented and the fees that would be paid to lawyers.

With the unexpected denial of Social Security disability benefits I was faced with two options. I could wait five years until I was sixty-five years of age and receive full benefits, or I could proceed with the appeal process. I did not think it would be wise to try and get through the next five years without health insurance, and since Medicare was the only insurance option available to me I opted to file an appeal.

As much as I dislike litigation I decided that it would be unwise to try to plow through what looked like a forest of bureaucratic red tape on my own. The local phone book listed three lawyers that specialized in Social Security litigation. Two of those lawyers would not consider my case until my appeal had been denied. It seemed to be a foregone conclusion that it would be denied. I went with the third lawyer who was willing to start at square one, beginning with my appeal.

On July 15, 1993 I found myself in a place and a situation that was both new and unexpected. I was in a lawyer's office about to sue an agency of the United States Government. The lawyer that I had selected turned out to be a two-person law firm that specialized in Social Security claims. I was met by the junior partner of the firm who assured me that I would eventually be successful because I was over sixty years of age. I signed a fee agreement that was approved by the Social Security Administration. It fixed the fee at "25% of the amount of past due benefits not to exceed $4000.00, whichever is less." Not very good grammar, but they made their point.

The agreement also had a clause that stated that they would not be paid unless they were successful in obtaining benefits. That clause was a virtual guarantee to me that I would receive full benefits. It seemed to be obvious that the attorneys would not have taken the case unless they were very sure that they would win and be paid for their services. After signing the agreement I was introduced to a legal clerk who would handle the paperwork.

The legal clerk turned out to be a very pregnant young lady who appeared to be ready to go into labor at any minute. She explained that because they were located in a relatively poor section of the city most of their clients were people trying to get benefits for a sickness or injury that prevented them from working. Compared to some of those cases my case was expected to be a slam-dunk.

The first order of business was for me to sign about a dozen form letters and documents that would be used as the case developed. The appeal process was so well defined that they knew exactly what correspondence would be received from the Social Security Administration, and they had a letter or document ready with the appropriate response. The letters and documents that I had signed were ready to be dated and mailed as needed. It would not be necessary for me to make another visit to their office.

About six weeks after my appeal was filed I received a letter from the State of Florida, Department of Labor and Employment Security, advising me that the Social Security Administration had passed my file to them to determine if I met "the requirements for disability benefits." They further stated that after reviewing my case they needed "more information about my condition." To obtain that information they had made an appointment for me with a doctor that they would "pay for from funds provided by Social Security." They included a list of things I should bring with me and things I should do. The list included the requirement that I should "bathe and wear clean clothing."

The doctor that they had selected was located in a walk-in clinic. After completing the usual paperwork I received a detailed physical examination. That examination seemed to have been designed to evaluate a person who was engaged in a job that required a lot of physical activity.

A few weeks after the examination I received a copy of his report which included the comment that I was "pleasant and cooperative." I took that to mean that some of his clients were neither pleasant nor cooperative, which probably explained the item about bathing and clean clothes. His conclusion stated that "the findings in my opinion do not reveal conclusively for total and permanent disability." I assumed that statement to be a "no" to my claim for disability benefits, but not a strong one.

On November 4, 1993 my appeal was denied with a form letter similar to the first denial. The key point in the denial was my failure to find the elusive "work which requires less physical effort." Things seemed to be right on track as we moved to the next phase. On November 23, 1993 we filed a request for a hearing before an Administrative Law Judge.

There was no further communication until September 2, 1994 when we received notification that a "wholly favorable decision can be issued without the necessity of a hearing." The pertinent points related to that decision were:

"The claimant continued working for a number of years, despite the diagnosis of Parkinson's disease. The medical evidence establishes the gradual increase in his complaints and symptomatology related to the disease. He finally became unable to continue engaging in substantial gainful activity as a mechanical engineer, having increased problems due to his hand tremor."

"The evidence supports a finding that he cannot perform his past relevant work as a mechanical engineer. The use of his hands was highly important to performing such work."

"The claimant was 60 years old on the date disability began, which is defined as closely approaching retirement age."

The outcome was exactly as predicted. All of the above facts were known when I filed for benefits in the spring of 1993. Yet to obtain benefits I had to wait a year and a half without health insurance, and I had to hire a lawyer. It is my understanding that all claimants for disability benefits, unless they are virtually basket cases, receive the same treatment.

A few weeks after the decision, I received a check from the Social Security Administration for past due benefits, less the lawyer's fee, which had been deducted from the total and paid directly to the lawyer. The only sure-fire winners in the appeal process are members of the legal profession. I suppose the Social Security Administration could also be considered a winner if a claimant expired during the appeal process.

With the completion of the move to Florida and the resolution of the problems with the Social Security Administration it was time to get back to the business of living with Parkinson's disease. There had been some drugs added to the Parkinson's mix around the turn of the century that were found to be helpful to some people, but there was nothing to challenge levodopa therapy as the primary medication for the treatment of the disease. My long established drug regimen was controlling my Parkinson's as well as could be expected, so there was no reason to consider using any of the new drugs.

After the demise of the adrenal transplant craze, neurosurgeons continued to pursue surgical solutions that would help control the debilitating effects of Parkinson's disease. Realizing that the day will come when drugs will no longer control my Parkinson's I felt that it was necessary for me to understand the surgical options that were available.

At the present time there are three types of surgery available for Parkinson's disease. The first surgery could be referred to as the procedure offered by…

PART NINE

The Last Resort: Neurosurgery

20. The Ablaters

To obtain an understanding of the benefits of a surgical procedure it is necessary to have a basic understanding of the various steps involved in that procedure. The following is a description of the basic steps involved in the procedure known as ablative surgery.

The dictionary defines ablation as destruction. Ablative surgery is therefore performed to destroy a part of the body that is impeding the proper functioning of the body. Ablative surgery related to the brain consists of locating a specific part of the brain that is malfunctioning and destroying, or ablating it.

Ablative surgery for Parkinson's disease was initiated in the nineteen-fifties when it was discovered that some areas of the brain that were damaged by the disease produced an abnormal chemical or electrical discharge. Researchers were able to determine the location of an abnormal discharge within the brain, but were unable to correct the problem at its source.

Some researchers believed that the abnormal discharge generated an abnormal signal that in turn disrupted the normal, harmonious operation of the brain. It was also believed that the destruction of an area of the brain that generated an abnormal signal allowed a more normal functioning of the rest of the brain.

The first target for ablative surgery, related to Parkinson's disease, was an area of the brain known as the globus pallidus. The procedure became known as a pallidotomy and was intended initially to reduce the tremor experienced by people with the disease. That procedure was followed in the nineteen-sixties by an ablative surgery that targeted an area of the brain known as the thalamus, in a procedure that became known as a thalamotomy. It was also intended to reduce tremor.

Surgery for both procedures is similar. The procedure begins when the surgeon numbs the scalp, which contains pain sensitive nerves, with a local anesthetic. A small hole is then drilled into the skull which exposes the underlying brain covering. This membrane also contains pain sensitive nerves, and is also numbed with a local anesthetic. The rest of the operation is painless because the brain itself does not have any pain-sensitive nerves. This allows the patient to be awake for the entire procedure.

The next step in the procedure is to insert a metallic probe, which functions as an electrode, through the brain covering into the brain. The probe is then directed past the numerous blood vessels that crisscross the brain, into the target area. Navigating the probe through the blood vessels is not without risk. Blood vessels could be ruptured and bleeding could occur. Bleeding could be minor, without consequences, or it could be major, resulting in paralysis or death.

After the probe has been correctly positioned it is heated to ablate the targeted area. The procedure is opposite handed in that the left side of the brain controls the right side of the body, and vice-versa. When the patient's opposite side tremor ceases the probe is removed. Heating of the probe causes brain tissue adjacent to the probe to swell, which in turn causes the ablated area to appear to be larger than its true size. When the swelling subsides it could reveal that the ablation was incomplete and the tremor could return.

It is generally accepted that because of complications such as swelling, most surgeons are unable to correctly determine the intensity and duration of the burn needed to permanently destroy a tremor. To avoid problems they often induce a smaller burn than might be needed because it is much safer to chance the return of the tremor than to risk the paralysis which could result from a larger burn.

Ablative surgery at best is very much a hit or miss proposition. The lack of control that the surgeon has over this procedure would appear to place the patient in a position where the degree of risk exceeds any anticipated reward.

I find it hard to believe that anybody with Parkinson's disease ever received any real benefit from this type of surgery. Some short term relief perhaps, but nothing permanent that would be worth the risk that is incurred by destroying a part of the brain. Michael J. Fox had a thalamotomy with little, if any, real benefit. His unmedicated and courageous appearances before the United States Congress were vivid demonstrations of Parkinson's disease out of control. His appearance on each occasion was devoid of any indication that he had received any benefit from his surgery.

With the memory of my cervical laminectomy still strong after all those years, I have a built-in aversion to surgery. I am afraid that I would need an iron clad guarantee of success before undergoing another procedure. With its present track record there is no way that I could ever consider ablative surgery for my Parkinson's disease. Apart from its history of little if any success, the thought of somebody probing around inside my head with a hot wire is more than I can handle.

In addition to the above concerns, ablative surgery does not correct the chemical imbalance within the brain of a person with Parkinson's disease. It does nothing to correct the loss of dopamine, which is the acknowledged cause of Parkinson's disease. It is difficult to understand how anyone could expect ablative surgery to benefit a person with the disease.

When comparing the three types of surgery currently available for Parkinson's disease, it should be noted that ablative surgery is the lowest cost option. The second procedure, the middle cost option, could be referred to as the procedure offered by…

21. The Transplanters

Transplantation surgery for Parkinson's disease involves the implanting of dopamine-producing cells into the brain of a person with Parkinson's. This is the same area of the brain that was the focal point of adrenal gland transplants in the nineteen-eighties. At that time it was determined that cells from the adrenal gland were unsuitable for transplantation. The difference with the surgery this time around is that the source of the cells has changed.

Dopamine-producing cells for transplantation surgery were taken from the patient's carotid body, which is a small cluster of dopamine producing cells that encircle the carotid artery in the neck. This procedure has had limited success primarily because there are not enough cells in the carotid body to achieve a successful implantation.

A more successful source of dopamine producing cells has been found in aborted human embryos. In this instance it has been demonstrated that embryo transplantation is "moderately beneficial to some patients, mostly those under sixty years of age."

"Moderately beneficial" is considerably less than a ringing endorsement of the procedure. "Mostly those under sixty" diminishes it even further. The biggest problem with this procedure is not its questionable performance, but the ethical questions surrounding the source of the transplantable cells.

It has been estimated that 80-90% of the transplanted cells will die during implantation because they fail to establish connections within the patient's brain. This means that at least four embryos are needed for each implantation.

It has been established that human embryos have to be harvested at between 9 and 12 weeks gestation because these are the only embryos that contain cells that can differentiate into dopamine producing cells. This creates a considerable supply problem because nearly all abortions are performed before the ninth week. The availability of suitable embryos is further complicated by the dissimilarity among embryos, and the necessary rejection of some embryos for viruses and other infectious agents that make them unsuitable for implantation.

A further complication in transplantation surgery is the unresolved issue regarding the use of immuno-suppressive drugs. These drugs are usually administered to patients to prevent the brain from rejecting the cells. Not all researchers believe in the necessity of using these drugs.

To overcome the problems encountered with the availability of human embryos researchers have turned to the possibility of using pig embryos as a source of cells. Pigs are immunologically close to humans. This means that an unlimited number of cells could be obtained from specially bred pig embryos. Research with pig embryos appears to be promising, however it should be noted that all new research has to look promising or it would never be funded in the first place. Realistically the possibility of getting a tissue match with a pig embryo is only a little better than finding a pot of gold at the end of a rainbow.

The risk factor associated with transplantation surgery is similar to ablation surgery. Bleeding could occur during the transplantation procedure. Paralysis and death are possible. While the results of ablative surgery are apparent almost immediately, the benefits of transplantation surgery will not be apparent for several months. The result will not be known until the new cells integrate themselves into the patient's brain.

Because of the problems involved with obtaining human embryos, and the less than acceptable results, it is highly unlikely that transplantation surgery will ever be a viable option for people with Parkinson's disease.

Having determined that the first two surgical options to alleviate Parkinson's disease appear to be unacceptable, we come to what could be considered as the main event. It is the most expensive option and could be referred to as the procedure offered by…

22. The Stimulators

The surgical procedure known as deep brain stimulation (DBS) consists of implanting an electrode into a part of the brain that has been identified as the source of an abnormal electrical discharge. In this regard it is similar to ablative surgery. The difference in the two procedures is that instead of destroying the region producing the abnormal discharge an electrical counter-current is introduced to block the abnormal current.

This is a significant improvement over ablative surgery. The first and most obvious improvement is that it does not destroy a portion of the brain. The second advantage over ablative surgery is that the magnitude of the counter-current can be adjusted to suit the needs of the patient, both initially and over the long term.

Deep brain stimulation surgery was initiated in the nineteen-eighties with the first successful implant in France in 1987. Since that date the procedure has been performed in many countries. While the procedure is not a cure for Parkinson's disease some of the implants have apparently been successful in improving the quality of life of the patient.

The surgical procedure for DBS is similar to ablative surgery in that holes are drilled in the skull of the patient. Electrodes are then implanted in the targeted area or areas of the brain. A wire from each electrode is routed under the skin and down the neck of the patient to a neurotransmitter that is mounted on the chest wall in much the same way that a cardiac pacemaker is installed. The neurotransmitter is turned on or off by an external magnet and programmed to meet the needs of the patient. It can be reprogrammed from time to time to control any changes that might occur in the condition of the patient.

At this time there are three target areas for DBS surgery. As in ablative surgery the thalamus and the globus pallidus are targeted because they are sources of abnormal electrical discharges. With DBS surgery a third and much more important area is also targeted. The subthalamic nucleus (STN) is a small area located below the thalamus that is believed to play a major role in controlling a lot of the problems encountered by people with Parkinson's disease.

It has been determined that DBS surgery of the thalamus controls only the tremor that is encountered by people with Parkinson's disease. For that reason the thalamus is rarely the target of DBS surgery.

On the other hand DBS surgery that targets the globus pallidus usually provides effective control of tremor and bradykinesia which is the slowness of movement related to Parkinson's disease. However DBS surgery of the globus pallidus is less effective in the control of problems related to walking, balance and dyskinesia.

DBS surgery that targets the STN has been found to be effective for nearly all of the major symptoms related to Parkinson's disease. This includes tremor, bradykinesia, rigidity, as well as problems with walking and balance. Improvement with dyskinesia has been significantly less than with the other symptoms. DBS surgery that targets the STN is the most difficult of the three procedures to perform. The STN is smaller than the other areas and is located beneath the thalamus. Because of its size and location it presents a more difficult target for the installation of an electrode.

It has been estimated that about 70 percent of the patients who undergo DBS surgery experience a significant improvement in the symptoms related to their Parkinson's disease. As with ablative surgery the risk of injury to blood vessels in the brain when installing electrodes is still a major concern for those involved with DBS surgery. There is also a potential problem with the wires from the electrodes, which could break or cause an infection.

Exposure to shortwave, microwave and ultrasound diathermy can cause heating of implanted electrodes, which could result in severe injury or death. Some devices such as theft detectors and screening devices at airports can turn neurotransmitters on or off. While it is relatively easy to avoid these potential problems, DBS surgery is still very much an imperfect solution to the problems associated with Parkinson's disease.

DBS surgery, like ablative surgery, does not generate any dopamine to correct the chemical imbalance in the brain. That is to say, it does nothing to correct the condition that is considered to be the root cause of the disease. DBS surgery is still a relatively new procedure and its long-term benefits have yet to be assessed. Considering the risks involved with the surgery and the experimental nature of the procedure, a reasonable person would be hard pressed to consider DBS surgery as a viable option for the treatment of Parkinson's disease.

If it does nothing else, the above review of the available surgical options destroys the popular notion that brain surgery is an exact science.

DBS surgery is seen by some as the only worthwhile surgical option for people with Parkinson's disease. To take advantage of the situation American entrepreneurship has once again risen to the occasion. Some time ago my Parkinson's support group received a visit from...

23. The Carpetbaggers

The dictionary defines a carpetbagger as "any promoter from the outside whose influence is resented." The term was coined as a contemptuous reference to opportunists who moved into the South to take advantage of the unsettled conditions after the Civil War. The modern day equivalent of a carpetbagger would be a person from another place who is setting up shop to peddle their wares on your turf.

Some time ago my Parkinson's support group was the recipient of a presentation by a representative of a manufacturer of neurotransmitters that are used in DBS surgery. The representative was a very energetic young lady who had recently joined the company. She began her presentation by stating that DBS surgery using their neurotransmitter was "not a cure for Parkinson's disease." That statement was followed by the admission that "it did not always work." That seemed like a somewhat unusual opening for a sales presentation, but it was not totally unexpected because DBS surgery is considered by many to be less than perfect. She was apparently clearing away the negative aspects of her product before getting into the meat of her sales pitch.

Her opening statements were followed by the disclosure that Michael J. Fox had declined DBS surgery. She explained that his decision was "a matter of choice." That was a very believable statement when you consider that a few years ago he had a part of his brain destroyed by an unsuccessful ablative surgery. It is difficult to find anything wrong with his decision.

With the negative issues put to rest she got into the positive aspects of her product. The gist of her presentation was that when the available drugs were no longer effective DBS surgery was the best treatment available. She reasoned that while her product did not cure Parkinson's disease it could be considered as a device that would put the disease in a holding pattern until a cure was found. When a cure was found the DBS equipment could simply be turned off. It is also difficult to find anything wrong with that statement, assuming that the negative long-term side effects of the surgery would be minimal.

The next item of interest was the revelation that the latest round of stem cell research for Parkinson's disease had failed to pass muster. The apparent removal of the only competing technology to DBS surgery meant that she represented the only game in town. She tried very hard to be very matter-of-fact when she made that statement, but the prospect of all those sales commissions was more than she could handle. Her voice broke just a tad as she spoke the words.

A ten-minute videotape was next on the agenda. It told the story of a middle-aged gentleman who was virtually immobilized by Parkinson's disease. The tape followed him through DBS surgery to a successful conclusion where he had regained almost complete mobility. To say that it was an impressive performance would be a huge understatement. It was more like a miracle.

The videotape also contained some footage of two officers of the company discussing the successful surgery that we had just seen. They were obviously quite pleased with the result. They were also very candid in stating that "we don't know why it works." That was hardly a ringing endorsement for their product and left me wondering if they really knew what they were doing. Always the cynic when it comes to miracles and near miracles, I immediately wondered what a follow-up tape of that gentleman would show if it were taken two or three years after his DBS surgery.

Near the end of her presentation she addressed some sales literature that she had distributed. It contained some success stories of middle aged people who had DBS products from her company implanted with very impressive results. It went on to identify people who may be candidates for their DBS products as "advanced levodopa-responsive Parkinson's patients with movement-related symptoms that cannot be controlled by drugs, and people who experience intolerable side effects from drugs." That statement was intended to establish DBS surgery as the next step for people with Parkinson's disease when their drug therapy starts to wear a little thin.

In the fine print on the back page of the sales literature was an item identified as "adverse events." It was probably prepared by their legal department because it listed just about everything that could go wrong. The more recognizable "adverse events related to the therapy, device, or procedure," were "stimulation not effective, cognitive disorders, dyskinesia, intracranial hemorrhage, cardiovascular events, seizures and respiratory events." The only thing that seemed to be missing from the list was an exclusion for earthquakes and other Acts of God. Nevertheless it did make the point that neurosurgery is a very risky business and they had taken the necessary steps to reduce their liability for "adverse events."

In closing she announced that a neurosurgeon who was very experienced in implanting DBS equipment manufactured by her company was relocating to our area. She alluded to his impressive track record of successful implants and assured us that he was one of the best. With the cost of DBS surgery now approaching six figures, she informed us that Medicare had recently approved DBS surgery for the treatment of Parkinson's disease in the State of Florida. This approval was probably a major factor in the neurosurgeon's decision to relocate to Florida.

It seems that people with Parkinson's disease have finally been commercialized. No longer will we be able to just fade away. We will be badgered to accept the risks associated with procedures like DBS surgery in the hope that it might work. It seems that the manufacturers of neurotransmitters and other people involved with DBS surgery are probably going to make a lot of money. However the number of people who will receive any real improvement to their Parkinson's could very well be a whole different story.

I have just about reached the end of my tale. Before blowing out the candle I feel it my duty to pass on some words of wisdom to the uninitiated. To complete this story I offer some…

PART TEN

Summation: Lessons Learned

24. Words of Wisdom

After more than twenty years in the trenches with Parkinson's disease I offer the following nuggets for living with the disease:

1. If your neurologist tells you that your resting tremor is the onset of essential tremor, get another opinion.
2. If your neurologist suggests that the calcium deposits inside your cervical vertebrae are the cause of your tremor and coordination problems, get another opinion.
3. Levodopa with carbidopa added as an inhibitor is the only drug that delivers dopamine to your brain. Use it wisely.
4. Exercise is the only activity that produces dopamine. Do it.
5. Why me? Never ask that question because there is no answer.
6. Parkinson's is a lonely battle, so join a support group to share the load.
7. Always keep your bodyweight slightly forward when standing or walking so that if you fall you will be able to use your hands to negotiate a soft landing.
8. To be a regular guy or gal, eat lots of fruit and lots of vegetables. Drink lots of water.

9. Be careful when you swallow because inhaling food or liquid into your lungs could lead to pneumonia, a condition you do not want to have to deal with.

Bibliography

The following publications were used in the preparation of this book:

Deprenyl: The Anti-Aging Drug by Alastair Dow

Surgery for Parkinson's Disease by Abraham Lieberman, M.D.

Parkinson's Disease. Hope Through Research. Published by the National Institute of Neurological Disorders and Stroke (NINDS)

Anatomy, Descriptive and Surgical by Henry Gray, F.R.S.

Report of the Presidential Commission on the Space Shuttle Challenger Accident (The Rogers Report)

Mayo Clinic Family Health Book David E. Larson, M.D., Editor-in-Chief

Bibliography

Appendix A – Notes on Exercising

Recommended types of exercise:

The goal of a person with Parkinson's is to have an exercise routine that will induce his or her brain to produce a little more dopamine than it would otherwise produce. The type of exercise routine and the level of intensity to accomplish that goal will vary from person to person. A successful exercise routine for people with Parkinson's comes down to finding a suitable type of exercise and an acceptable level of intensity.

The following types of exercise are recommended for people with Parkinson's disease. They are listed in order of preference. An individual with Parkinson's should select the best option for his or her situation.

- Progressive resistance exercise using free weights i.e. bar bells and dumb bells. See Appendix E for a basic weight training program using dumb bells.
- Progressive resistance exercise using machines that have pulleys or levers to raise a stack of weights.
- Bicycle riding if your coordination, balance and level of fitness allow you to exercise at an acceptable level of intensity.
- Rowing if you have the facilities.

- Swimming if you have the facilities.
- Running if you do not have joint or respiratory problems.
- Stationary bicycle with adjustable resistance.
- Stationary rowing machine with a sliding seat that will allow you to exercise your legs as well as your arms.
- Striding or fast walking.
- Anything else that increases respiration and produces perspiration.

Recommendations for performing an exercise routine:

- Join an exercise group if possible, because exercising alone is probably the most boring activity in the world.
- Warm-up properly before beginning an exercise routine.
- Perform all exercises correctly, especially if you are using free weights.
- Work out at least three days per week. If possible, workout six or even seven days per week.
- Never over-exercise. The only pain you should accept is a low-level muscle pain. Events such as joint pain, chest pain or breathing problems should not be accepted without professional guidance.

My present exercise routine:

- Exercise with free weights and machines for about 45 minutes, 3 times a week.
- Run a distance of about one mile, 3 or 4 times a week

Appendix B – Notes on Medications

With the knowledge that all drugs for the treatment of Parkinson's lose their effectiveness over time, the goal of a person with the disease is to extend the useful life of levodopa therapy by minimizing the rate at which it is used. That is accomplished by using the drugs that are approved for the treatment of Parkinson's disease and establishing the lowest effective daily dosage of levodopa. To achieve this goal it is necessary to find a physician who will buy into the low dosage concept and work with you to find the appropriate medications.

- If possible, all medications should be taken on an empty stomach to maximize absorption into the bloodstream.
- If you are using generic drugs, stay with the same manufacturer to avoid the variations in strength that exist between the manufacturers of generic drugs.
- If you are going to eat a protein rich meal, levodopa should be taken at least one hour before that meal.
- If you are taking deprenyl, wine and cheese should be avoided.

My daily medication regimen:

½ - 25/100 mg carbidopa/levodopa tablet 4 times a day

1 – 100 mg symmetrel capsule 2 times a day

1 – 5 mg deprenyl tablet 1 time a day

Appendix C – Most Common Symptoms of Parkinson's Disease:

Tremor

The most common symptom of Parkinson's disease. It is the uncontrolled shaking of body parts. It usually begins with the hands before advancing to the arms and legs.

Bradykinesia

Slowness of movement. Also difficulty in beginning a movement and changing the direction of a movement.

Dyskinesia

The uncontrolled movement of body parts usually beginning with the arms.

Rigidity

Increased stiffness of movement caused by the loss of coordination between counteracting muscles. Movement is impeded so that it resembles a ratcheting motion.

Appendix D – Basic Medications for Parkinson's Disease:

Carbidopa/Levodopa

Levodopa with carbidopa added as an inhibitor is the only medication that replaces some of the dopamine that has been lost to the disease. It is marketed under the trade or brand name of sinemet. In an attempt to confuse the issue the drug manufacturers have chosen to market the generic for sinemet under the name of carbidopa and levodopa.

Symmetrel

Developed as an anti-flu drug. It was found to reduce tremor in some Parkinson's patients. Its generic is marketed under the name of amantadine.

Deprenyl

Developed in Europe as an anti-aging drug. In some cases, when it is used with levodopa, it has been found to prolong the useful life of levodopa. It is marketed under the trade or brand name of eldepryl. Its generic is marketed under the name of selegiline.

Appendix E – The Daily Dozen

I have selected twelve basic weight training exercises for people with Parkinson's disease. All of these exercises were selected to be performed by a person who is not athletic and whose balance is impaired. People with unimpaired balance could pursue a more aggressive routine.

A person who has physical problems, other than Parkinson's, should obtain the approval of an appropriate health care professional before attempting this or any exercise program.

The only exercise equipment that you need for these basic exercises is a pair of adjustable plate loaded dumb bells. These dumb bells should have plates that range in size from about a pound and a quarter to ten pounds.

When exercising with dumb bells you should wear rubber soled shoes that are flexible. Clothing should be loose enough to allow unrestricted movement.

All exercises should be performed initially without dumb bells to become familiar with the various movements. A person who is unable to perform an exercise movement correctly without dumb bells should not attempt to use that exercise.

The dumb bells should then be loaded to determine the starting weight to be used for each exercise. A starting weight should be the heaviest weight that can be easily raised for eight repetitions. To monitor your progress the weight used in each exercise should be recorded on a chart. See Appendix F for a typical chart.

While it is desirable to have the same weights on each end of a dumb bell it is acceptable to overload one end. This will allow you a greater range in the weight of the loaded dumb bells. When a dumb bell is overloaded on one end it should be grasped with the thumb near the heavy end. Some exercises may require a weight that is less than the weight of the unloaded dumb bell. If that happens perform the exercise holding a single plate of the correct weight.

The starting weight should be increased when an exercise can be performed easily for twelve repetitions. Not all exercises will have their weights increased at the same time. Some exercises, usually those using heavier weights, can sometimes be increased after a few weeks. Other exercises may require months. Eventually all of the exercises will reach a point where a weight increase will not be possible. At that time a maintenance phase will begin where exercises will not produce gains in strength but should still retard the advance of Parkinson's disease.

These exercises can be performed at just about any time of the day. The only recommended exception would be immediately after eating, when the food is being digested.

Breathing is important when weight training. Air should be inhaled when the weight is being lowered and exhaled slowly when the weight is being raised.

Weight training for Parkinson's disease should be performed at least three times a week. Unfortunately there is no free lunch with Parkinson's so that on the days when you do not do the daily dozen you should be engaged in some other physical activity.

The twelve dumb bell exercises that I selected are illustrated on the following pages. The order in which they are shown is the order in which they could be performed. While it is desirable to do all of the selected exercises, your Parkinson's condition will benefit if you do less than the dozen. If there are exercises that you cannot do it is recommended that you repeat some that you can do, for a total of twelve exercises.

E.1 Forward Bend

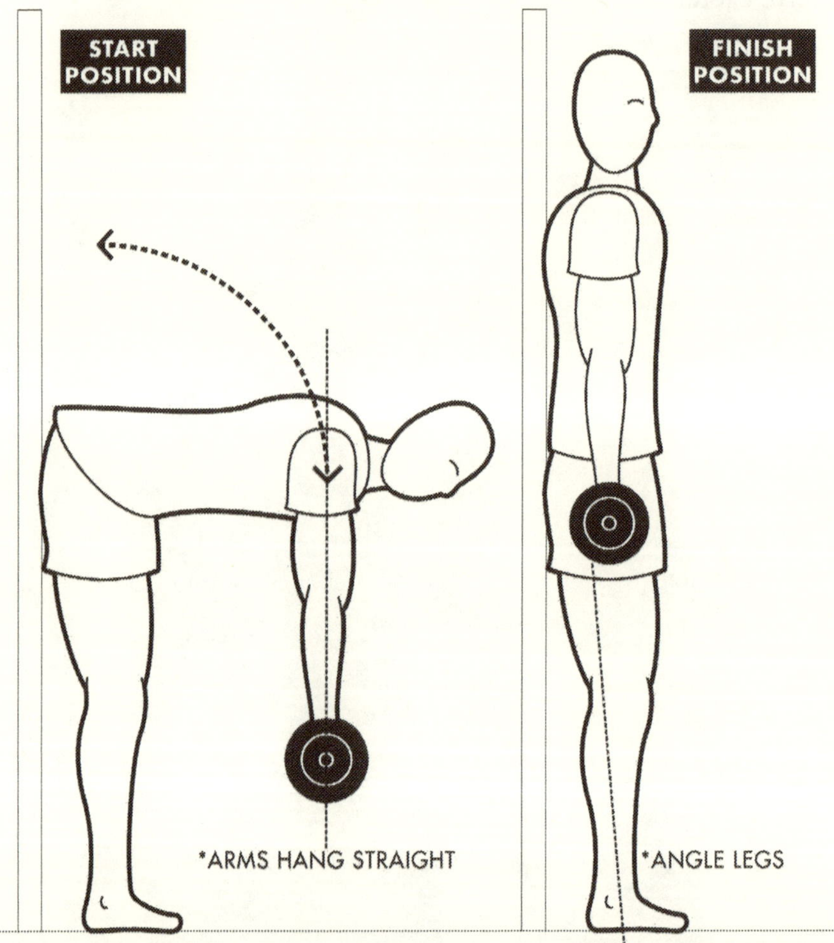

Grasp a dumb bell in each hand and stand with your back leaning against a wall. With your back and arms straight bend forward until your back is parallel to the floor. Your buttocks must remain in contact with the wall and your arms must hang straight at all times during this exercise.

•

Raise the dumb bells by returning to a standing position with your back against the wall.

•

Perform the exercise for a total of eight repetitions.

E.2 Toe Raise

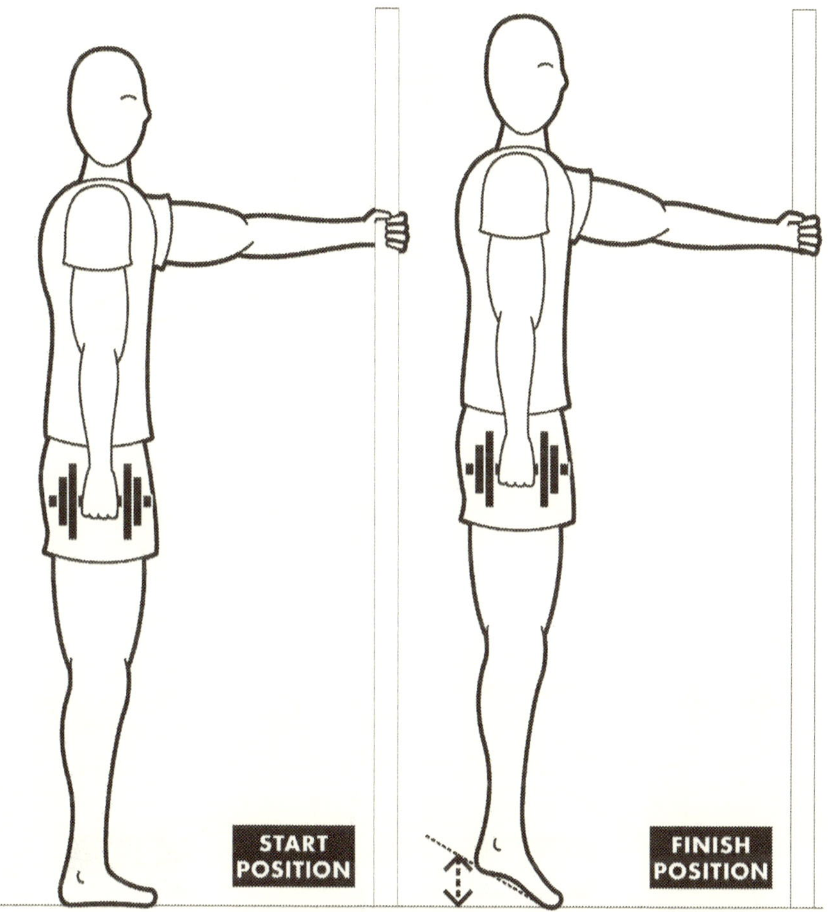

Grasp a dumb bell in your right hand and stand with your right arm hanging straight. Hold onto a door frame or some other vertical support with your left hand.

•

With your right arm hanging straight use your calf muscles to raise your body as high as possible by standing on your toes. Relax your calf muscles to lower your body to the starting position.

•

Perform the exercise for a total of eight repetitions.

•

Grasp the dumb bell in the left hand and repeat the exercise left-handed for eight repetitions.

E.3 Deep Knee Bend

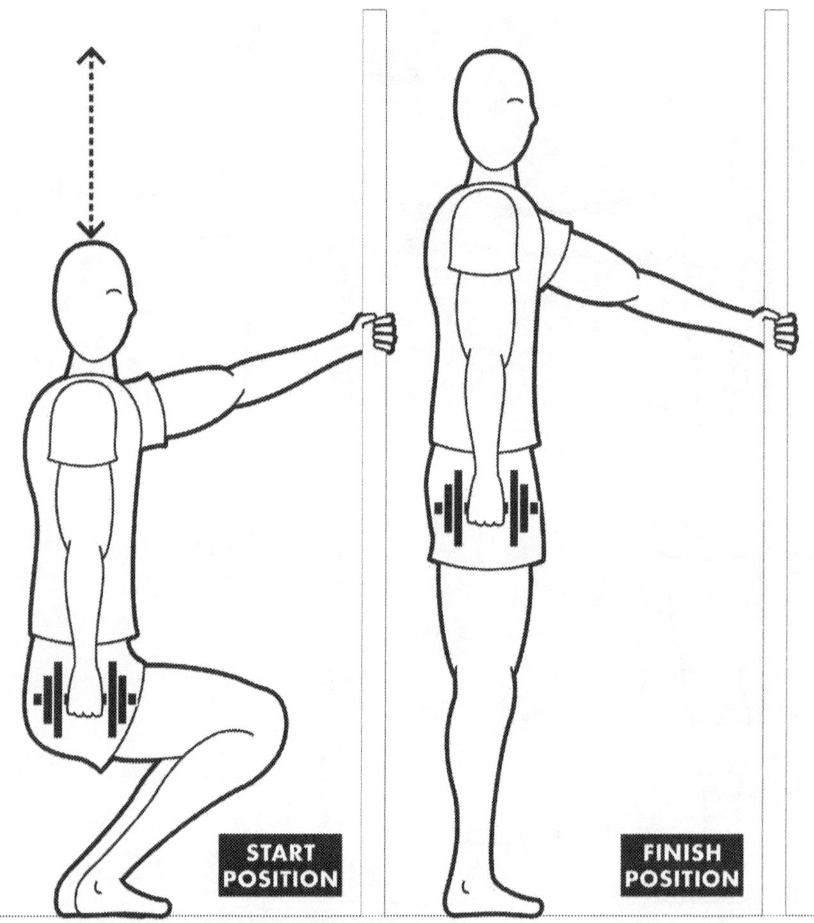

Grasp a dumb bell in your right hand and stand with your right arm hanging straight. Hold onto a door frame or some other vertical support with your left hand.

•

With the dumb bell in your hand and your right arm hanging straight lower your body to a full squat position. Raise the dumb bell by returning your body to a standing position.

•

Perform the exercise for a total of eight repetitions.

•

Grasp the dumb bell in your left hand and repeat the exercise left-handed for eight repetitions.

E.4 Biceps Curl

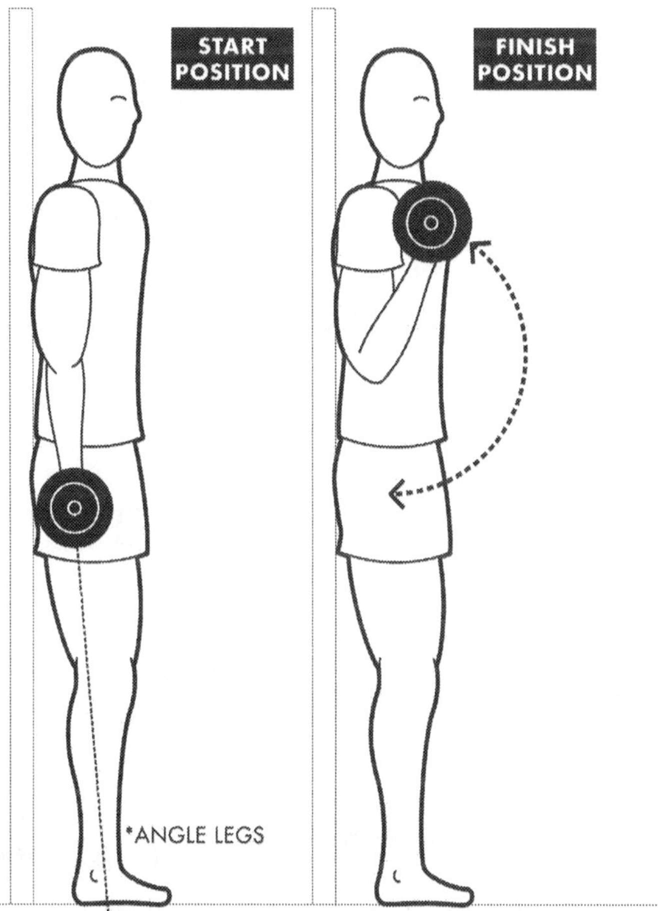

Grasp a dumb bell in each hand and stand with your back flat against a wall. Your arms should be hanging straight and the palms of your hands should be facing forward.

•

With the backs of your upper arms in contact with the wall raise both dumb bells as high as possible. Lower the dumb bells until your arms are straight.

•

Perform the exercise for a total of eight repetitions.

E.5 Triceps Extension

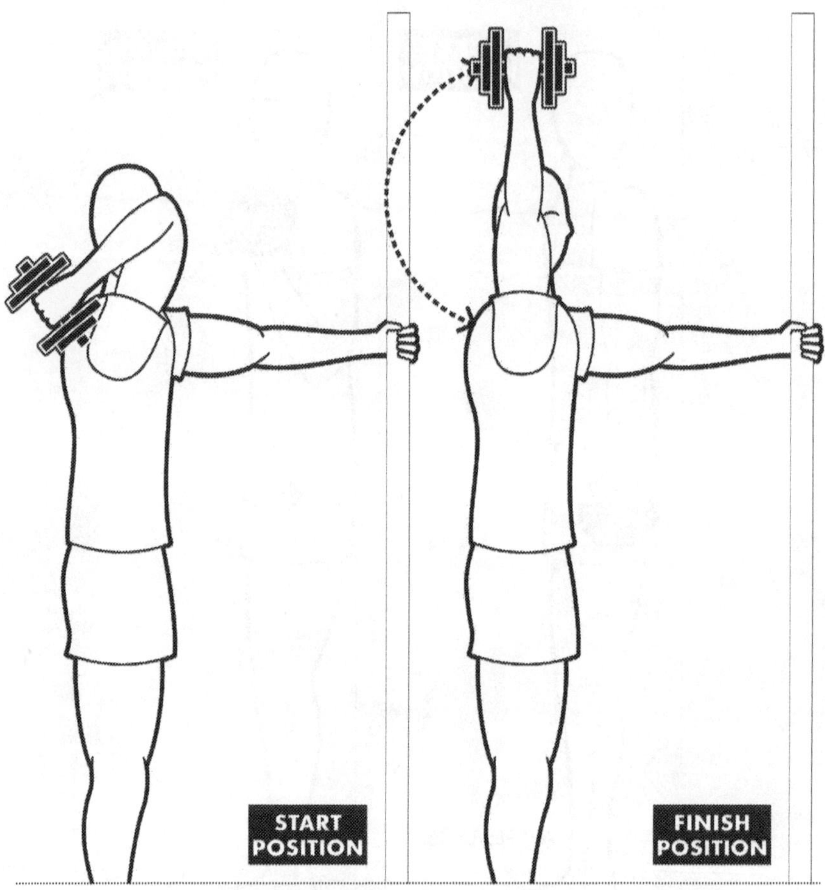

Grasp a dumb bell in your right hand. Stand with your right arm fully bent with the elbow raised to the maximum height above your head. Hold onto a door frame or some other vertical support with your left hand.

•

Raise the dumb bell vertically until your right arm is straight. Lower the dumb bell to the starting position.

•

Perform the exercise for a total of eight repetitions.

•

Grasp the dumb bell in your left hand and repeat the exercise left-handed for eight repetitions.

E.6 Press

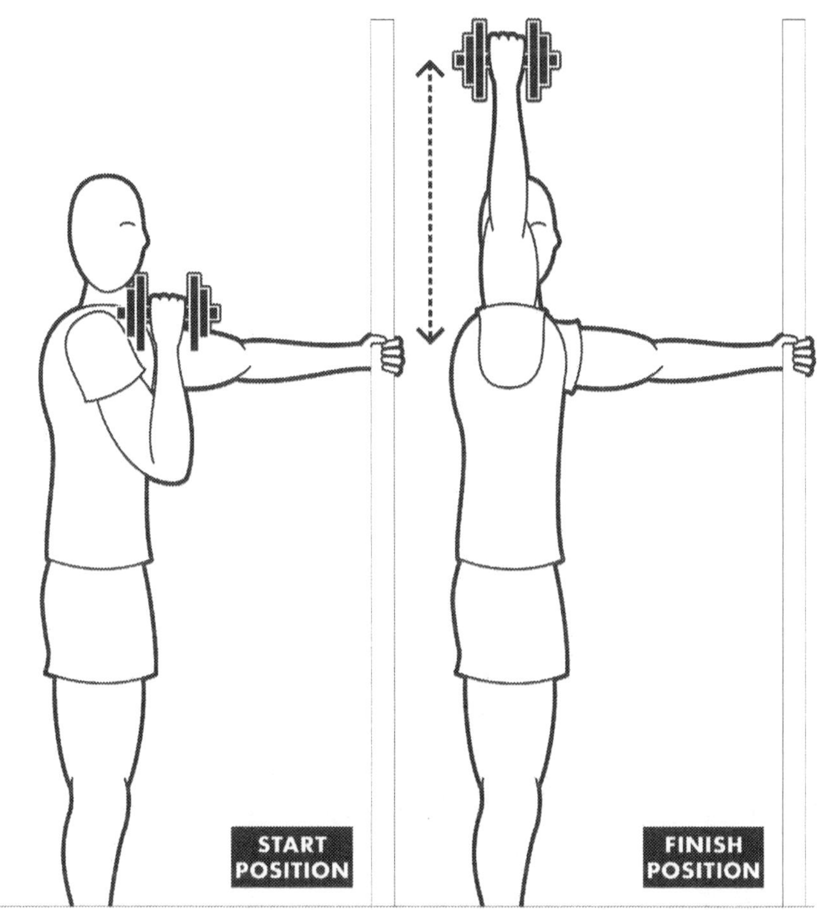

Grasp a dumb bell in your right hand and stand with your right arm fully bent and the dumb bell at shoulder height. Hold onto a door frame or some other vertical support with your left hand.

•

Raise the dumb bell as high as possible by straightening your right arm. Lower the dumb bell to the starting position.

•

Perform the exercise for a total of eight repetitions.

•

Grasp the dumb bell in your left hand and perform the exercise left-handed for eight repetitions.

E.7 Rowing Motion

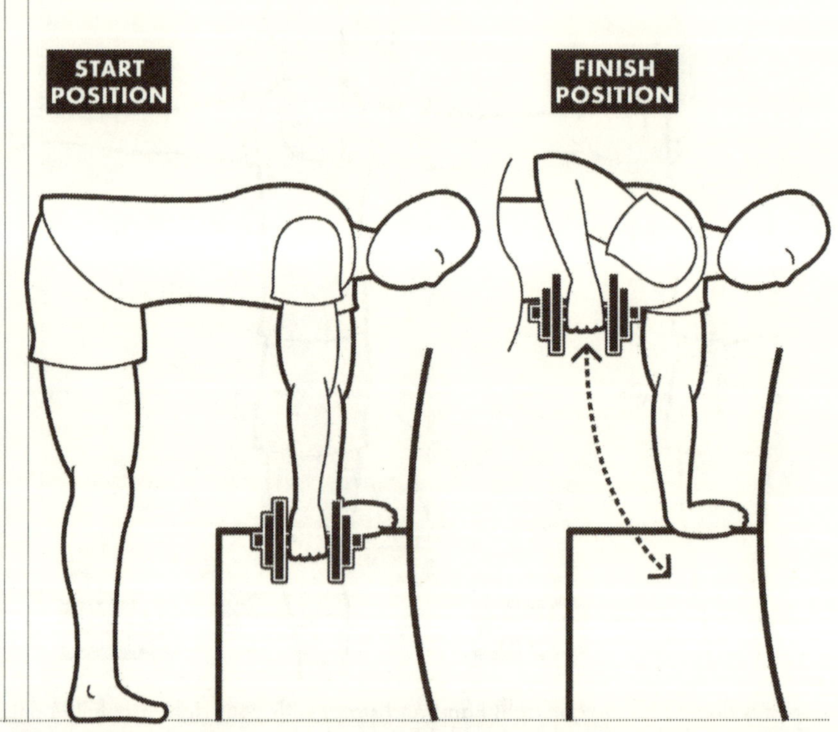

Grasp a dumb bell in your right hand and bend forward at the hips until your back is straight and horizontal. Hold onto a chair or some other horizontal support with your left hand to support your upper body. Your right arm should be hanging straight holding the dumb bell.

•

Raise the dumb bell until it contacts your rib cage. Lower the dumb bell to straight arm.

•

Perform the exercise for a total of eight repetitions.

•

Grasp the dumb bell with your left hand and repeat the exercise left-handed for eight repetitions.

E.8 Upright Rowing

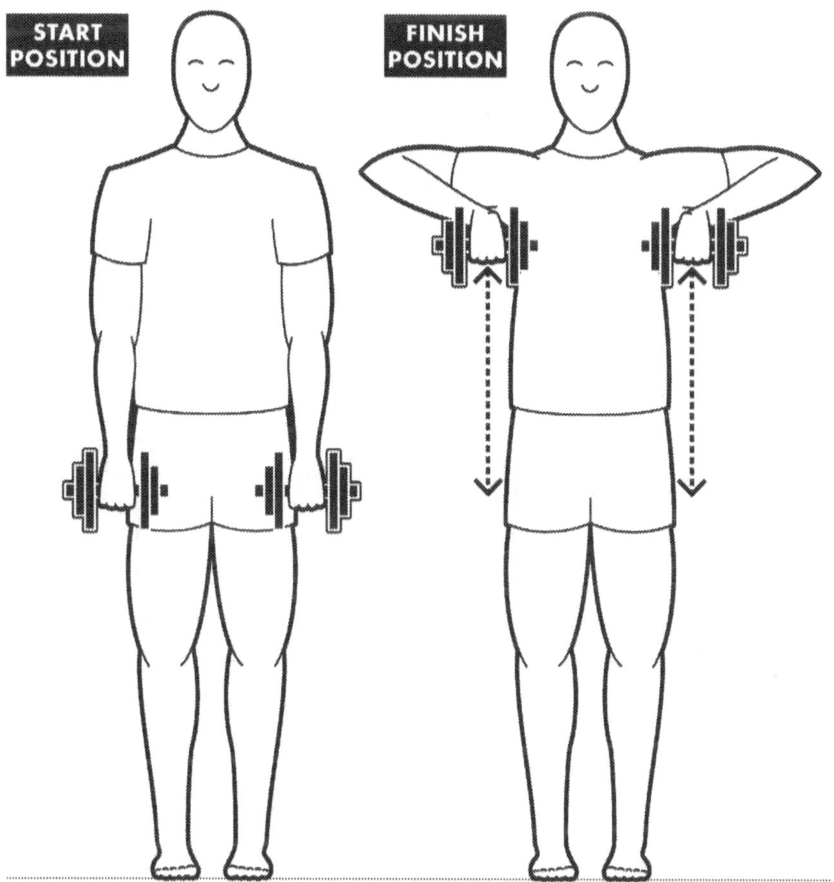

Grasp a dumb bell in each hand and stand with your back leaning against a wall. Your arms should be hanging straight and the palms of your hands should be facing backward.

•

With your back and shoulders in contact with the wall raise both dumb bells to shoulder height. Lower the dumb bells until your arms are straight.

•

Perform the exercise for a total of eight repetitions.

E.9 Shoulder Shrug

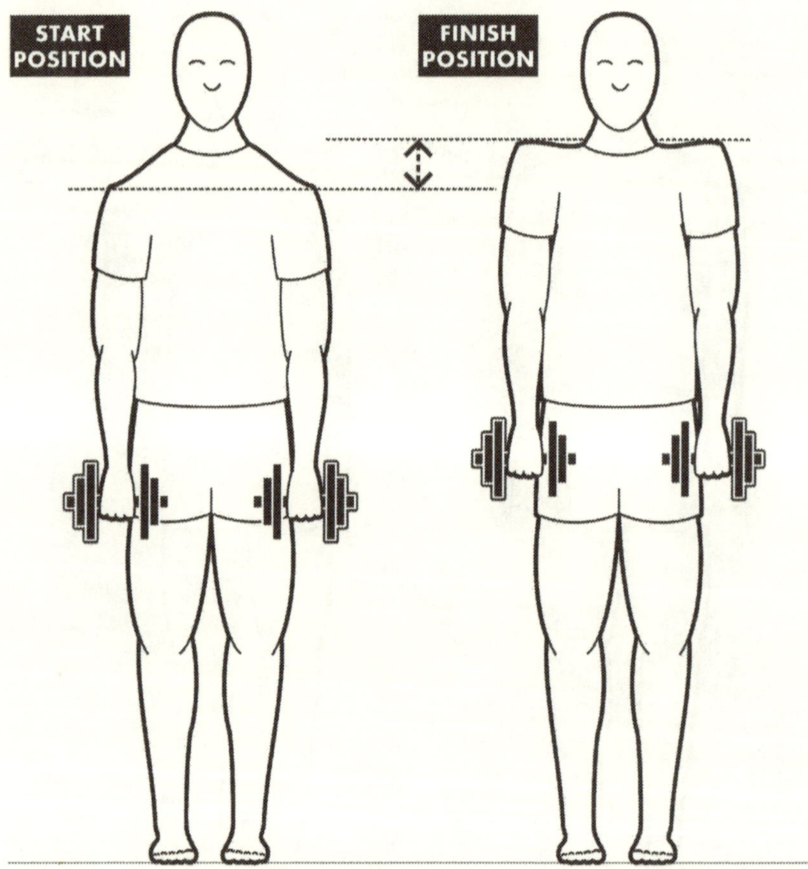

Grasp a dumb bell in each hand and stand with your back leaning against a wall. Your arms should be hanging straight and the palms of your hands should be facing backward. Your shoulders should hang as low as possible.

•

With your arms straight and your back in contact with the wall raise the dumb bells by raising your shoulders as high as possible.
Lower your shoulders to the starting position.

•

Perform the exercise for a total of eight repetitions.

E.10 Front Raise

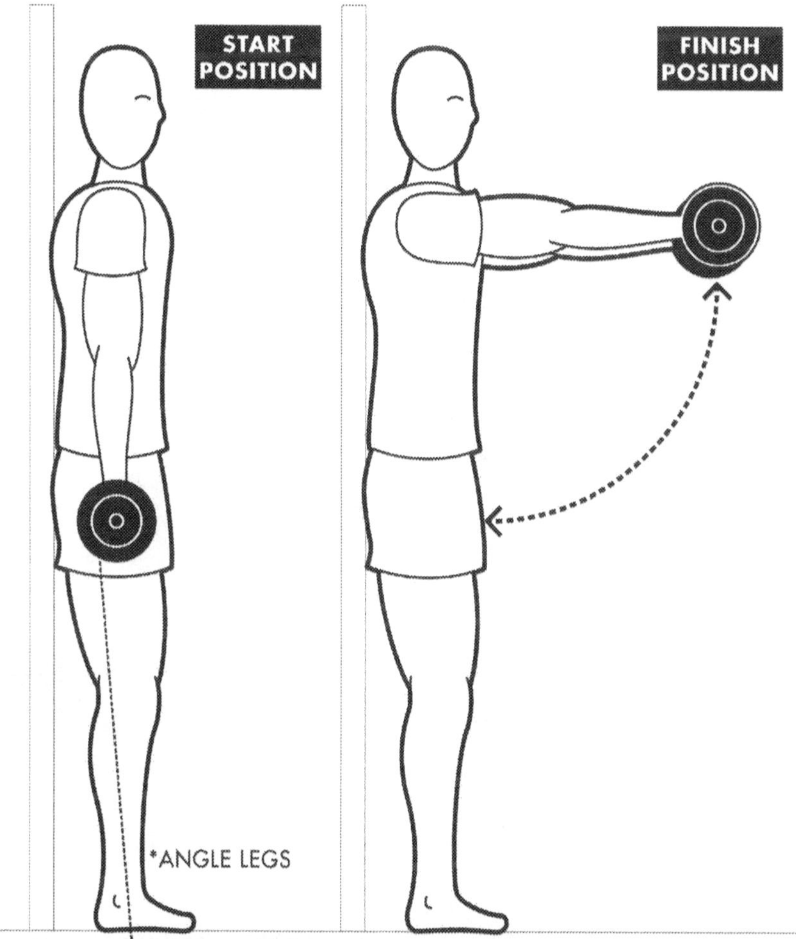

Grasp a dumb bell in each hand and stand with your back leaning against a wall. Your arms should be hanging straight and the palms of your hands should be facing backward.

•

With your arms straight and your back in contact with the wall raise both dumb bells directly in front of you until your arms are parallel to the floor. Lower the dumb bells to the starting position.

•

Perform the exercise for a total of eight repetitions.

E.11 Lateral Raise

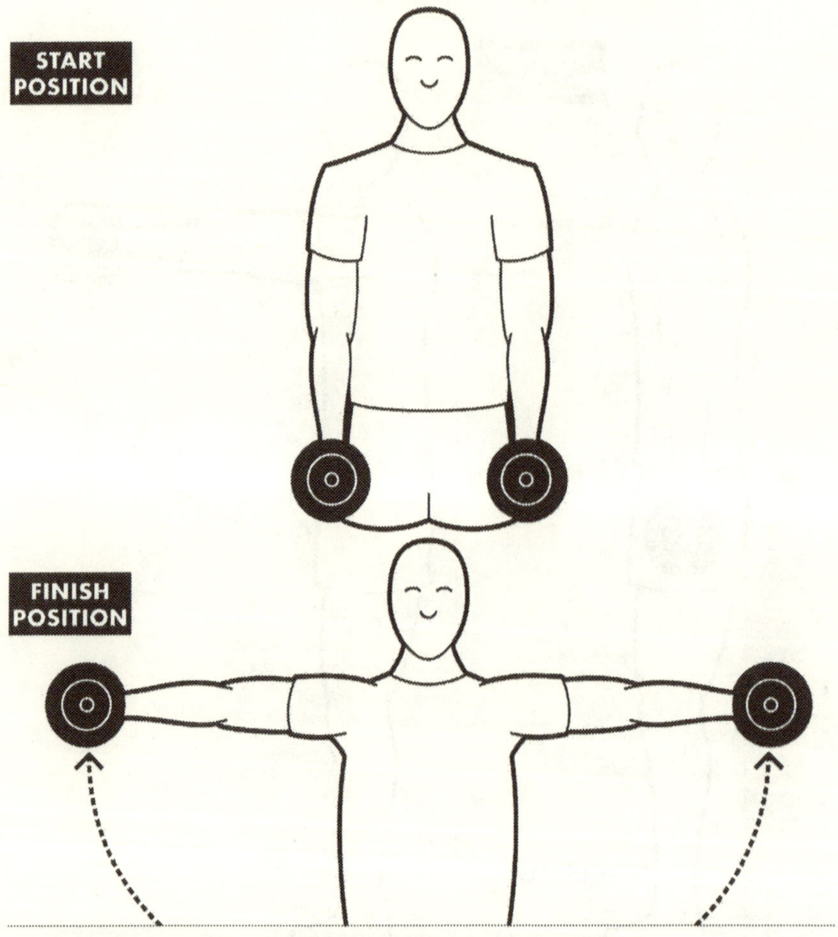

Grasp a dumb bell in each hand and stand with your back leaning against a wall. Your arms should be hanging straight and the palms of your hands should be facing each other.

•

With your arms straight and your back in contact with the wall raise both dumb bells sidewise until your arms are parallel to the floor. Lower the dumb bells to the starting position.

•

Perform the exercise for a total of eight repetitions.

E.12 Bent-over Lateral

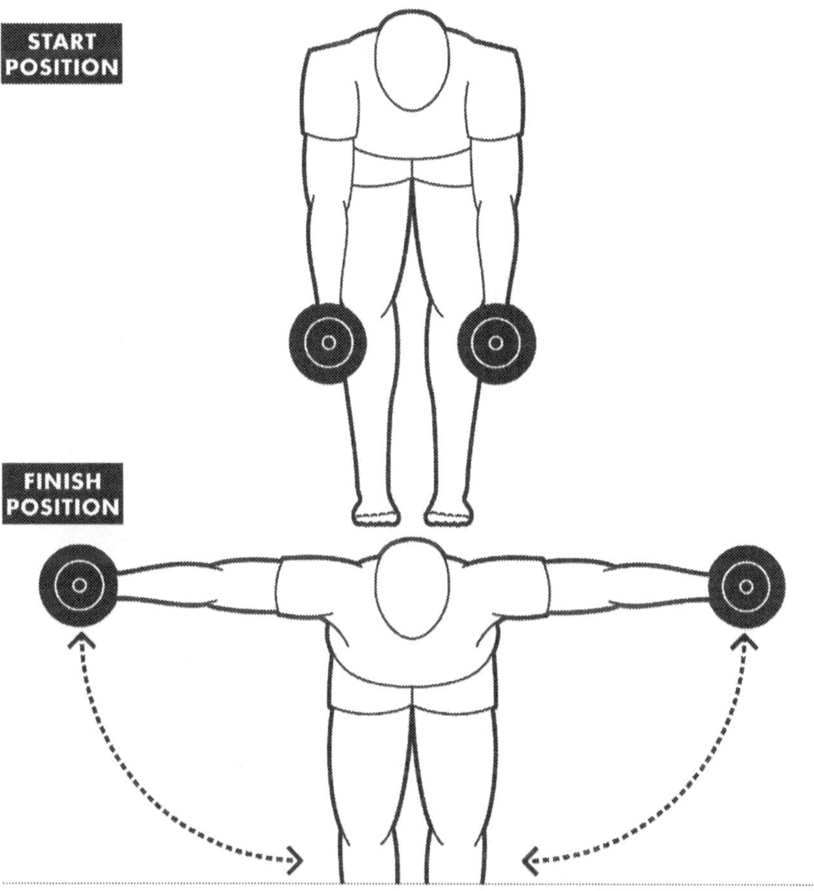

Grasp a dumb bell in each hand and stand with your buttocks leaning against a wall. Your back should be straight and parallel to the floor. Your arms should be hanging straight and the palms of your hands should be facing each other.

•

With your arms straight and your buttocks in contact with the wall raise both dumb bells sidewise until your arms are parallel to the floor. Lower the dumb bells to the starting position.

•

Perform the exercise for a total of eight repetitions.

Appendix F – Performance Chart

Performance Chart

EXERCISES	START WT.	WT. INCREASES				FINAL WT.
E.1 FORWARD BEND						
E.2 TOE RAISE						
E.3 DEEP KNEE BEND						
E.4 BICEPS CURL						
E.5 TRICEPS EXT.						
E.6 PRESS						
E.7 ROWING						
E.8 UPRIGHT ROW						
E.9 SHRUG						
E.10 FRONT RAISE						
E.11 LATERAL RAISE						
E.12 BENT OVER LATERAL						

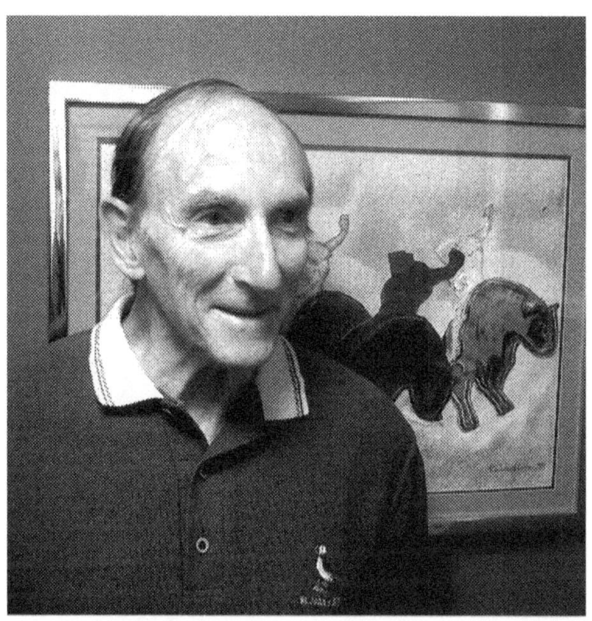

About the Author

Wilf Curren was born in St. John's, Newfoundland in 1932. He grew up during World War II when the City was home port to some of the warships that were engaged in what became known as the Battle of the Atlantic. He has vivid memories of those years when St. John's was virtually an armed camp, a constant reminder that the war was real and not very far away.

In 1951 he began weight training which became an activity that he has pursued for nearly all of his life. In 1955 he earned a degree in Mechanical Engineering from McGill University in Montreal. In 1963 he relocated to San Francisco's Sunset District, not too far from the corner of Haight and Ashbury. That location provided a ringside view of the cultural revolution that exploded in the turbulent Sixties.

After working at various locations in California and Texas he retired to Florida in 1993.

www.ingramcontent.com/pod-product-compliance
Lightning Source LLC
Chambersburg PA
CBHW030006190526
45157CB00014B/829

* 9 7 8 1 4 2 5 9 0 1 8 5 1 *